EXERCISES IN ULTRASONOGRAPHY:

AN INTRODUCTION TO NORMAL STRUCTURE AND FUNCTIONAL ANATOMY

D1573084

EXERCISES IN ULTRASONOGRAPHY:

AN INTRODUCTION TO NORMAL STRUCTURE AND FUNCTIONAL ANATOMY

REVA ARNEZ CURRY, PhD, RT(R), RDMS

Assistant Professor and Program Coordinator
Diagnostic Medical Sonography
Department of Diagnostic Imaging
Thomas Jefferson University College of Allied Health Sciences
Philadelphia, Pennsylvania

BETTY BATES TEMPKIN, BA, RT(R), RDMS

Ultrasound Consultant
Formerly, Clinical Director
Diagnostic Medical Sonography Program
Hillsborough Community College
Tampa, Florida

W.B. SAUNDERS COMPANY

A Division of Harcourt Brace & Company

Philadelphia, London, Toronto, Montreal, Sydney, Tokyo

W.B. SAUNDERS COMPANY
A Division of Harcourt Brace & Company

The Curtis Center
Independence Square West
Philadelphia, Pennsylvania 19106

EXERCISES IN ULTRASONOGRAPHY: An Introduction to Normal
Structure and Functional Anatomy   ISBN 0-7216-4962-9

Printed in the United States of America.

Last digit is the print number: 9   8   7   6   5   4   3   2   1

CONTRIBUTORS

REVA ARNEZ CURRY, PhD, RT(R), RDMS

Assistant Professor and Program Coordinator, Diagnostic Medical Sonography, Department of Diagnostic Imaging, Thomas Jefferson University College of Allied Health Sciences, Philadelphia, Pennsylvania

The Pancreas; The Urinary System; Appendices: Ultrasound Documents Related to Patient Examination; Patient Chart Information: Medical/Surgical Assembly Order

MARILYN DICKERSON, BS, RDMS

Instructor and Program Director, Diagnostic Medical Sonography Program, Emory University School of Medicine, Atlanta, Georgia

The Liver; The Gastrointestinal System

MICHAEL C. FOSS, MEd, RDMS, RVT

Associate Professor of Allied Health Sciences, Director, Sonography Program, Department of Allied Health Sciences, Rochester Institute of Technology College of Science, Rochester, New York

The Biliary System; The Pancreas

DANIEL HAGAN, RT(R), RDMS

Program Director, El Paso Community College, El Paso, Texas

Body Systems

FELICIA M. JONES, BS, RDMS, RVT

Program Director, Diagnostic Medical Sonography, Tidewater Community College, Virginia Beach, Virginia

The Spleen; Breast Sonography; Introduction to Ultrasound of Human Disease

MICHAEL J. KAMMERMEIER, BSRT, RDMS, RVT

Sonographer, Pennsylvania Hospital, Philadelphia, Pennsylvania

The Male Pelvis

ALEXANDER LANE, PhD

Coordinator of Anatomy and Physiology, Triton College, River Grove, Illinois

Anatomy Layering and Sectional Anatomy

WAYNE C. LEONHARDT, BA, RT, RDMS, RVT

Staff Sonographer and Clinical Instructor, Summit Medical Center, Oakland; Faculty, Foothill College, Los Altos; Ultrasound Program; Consultant for Ultrasound Education Program Development, Los Altos, California

Thyroid and Parathyroid Glands

HEATHER LEVY, BS, RT(R)

Sonographer/Radiographer, Memorial Sloan-Kettering Cancer Center, New York, New York

Appendices: Ultrasound Documents Related to Patient Examination; Ultrasound Instrumentation; Film Processing; Patient Chart Information: Medical/Surgical Assembly Order

MAUREEN E. McDONALD, BS, RDMS, RDCS

Instructor of Echocardiography, Ultrasound Diagnostic School, Philadelphia; Staff Echocardiographer, Thomas Jefferson University Hospital, Philadelphia, Pennsylvania

Adult Echocardiography

VIVIE M. MILLER, BA, BS, RDMS, RDCS

Clinical Instructor, Department of Pediatrics, Section of Pediatric Cardiology, Medical College of Georgia, Augusta, Georgia

Pediatric Echocardiography

MARSHA M. NEUMYER, BS, RVT

Instructor of Surgery, Pennsylvania State University College of Medicine, Hershey; Technical Director, Vascular Studies Section, Department of Surgery, The Milton S. Hershey Medical Center, Hershey, Pennsylvania

Vascular Technology

JERRY PEARSON, MSA, RDMS

Director of Diagnostic Radiology, University Hospital, Oregon Health Sciences University, Portland, Oregon

The Abdominal Aorta; The Inferior Vena Cava; The Portal Venous System

M. NATHAN PINKNEY, BS

Imaging Consultant, Sonicor Inc., West Point, Pennsylvania; Clinical Instructor, Diagnostic Medical Sonography, Department of Diagnostic Imaging, Thomas Jefferson University College of Allied Health Sciences, Philadelphia, Pennsylvania

Physics; Instrumentation

BRIAN A. SCHLOSSER, BS, RDMS

Staff Sonographer, Children's Hospital of the King's Daughters, Norfolk, Virginia

The Neonatal Brain

G. WILLIAM SHEPHERD, PhD, RDMS, RVT

Clinical Instructor and Staff Ultrasonographer, Frankford Hospital, Philadelphia, Pennsylvania

The Urinary System; First Trimester Obstetrics; Second and Third Trimester Obstetrics; Obstetric Sonography/Special Situations

BETTY BATES TEMPKIN, BA, RT(R), RDMS

Ultrasound Consultant; Formerly Clinical Director Diagnostic Medical Sonography Program, Hillsborough Community College, Tampa, Florida

Anatomy Layering and Sectional Anatomy; The Pancreas; The Urinary System; Your First Scanning Experience

DEBORAH D. WERNEBURG, MBA, RDMS

Lecturer in Diagnostic Medical Sonography, Department of Diagnostic Imaging, College of Allied Health Sciences, Thomas Jefferson University Hospital, Philadelphia, Pennsylvania

The Female Pelvis

CONTENTS

INSTRUCTIONS FOR STUDENTS

The purpose of this manual is to assist you in studying concepts presented in the textbook ULTRASONOGRAPHY: AN INTRODUCTION TO NORMAL STRUCTURE AND FUNCTIONAL ANATOMY. The following are suggestions which may help you.

1. Pay attention to the key words and objectives. The key words are highlighted in the text to guide you on what is important. Keep the objectives in mind as you read the chapter.

2. Notice how most chapters are divided into main sections, including Location, Anatomy, Physiology, Sonographic Appearance, and Reference Charts. You may want to divide your reading by sections. For example, one evening you may read the Location and Gross Anatomy sections. The next evening, you might read the Physiology and Sonographic Appearance sections. We suggest you finish reading or studying an entire section before ending your study time. That way, you can pick up with a new concept the next time you study.

3. The Student Manual contains review questions designed to test you at a basic level on your ability to retain information you've just read. How well you answer these questions is an indicator of your comprehension. (The answers are located in the back of the manual so you can test and grade yourself.) The next step will be for you to get very comfortable with the material. Read other textbooks in the library and increase your knowledge on what we've presented.

4. This manual contains unlabeled images and illustrations from every chapter in the textbook to test your comfort level with sonograms and identifying anatomy. Make sure you understand the images which have been presented for you. Can you identify structures without labels? Do you know how to describe them? If you're still confused about the images presented here, go back and reread the section in the textbook. We encourage you to color the structures on the illustrations to better differentiate the anatomy.

5. A protocol for an abdominal aorta examination is included to help you with your first scanning experience. Study the images, illustrations, and directions carefully as you begin scanning.

6. Make sure you understand which things in the text are important *to your instructor*. Think of these as guidelines. Write these guidelines down and refer to them as you study. This technique should help you prepare for major tests on the material.

Sonography is an exciting and challenging profession; we wish you the best in your career.

Chapter 1

PHYSICS

REVIEW QUESTIONS

1. What is the primary difference between x-rays and ultrasound energy?

a. x-rays are ionizing and sound is electromagnetic

b. sound is mechanical

c. sound can travel through a vacuum

d. ultrasound is electromagnetic

2. Which of the following frequencies is not typically used for medical diagnostic ultrasound?

a. 100 kHz

b. 2.25 MHz

c. 3.5 MHz

d. 5.0 MHz

3. What determines the velocity of sound in a material?

a. stiffness and density

b. stiffness and frequency

c. density and intensity

d. density and frequency

4. What is the velocity of sound in human soft tissue?

a. 1540 mm per second

b. 1.54 mm per second

c. 1540 meters per microsecond

d. 1540 meters per second

5. What is a typical pulse repetition frequency in a diagnostic ultrasound system?

a. 1 MHz

b. 100 Hz

c. 1000 Hz

d. 1000 kHz

6. What does a backing material provide when used in a pulse-echo ultrasound transducer?

a. improved lateral resolution

b. damping

c. focusing

d. impedance matching

7. If the transducer frequency is doubled,

a. the period is doubled

b. the period is halved

c. the period is the same

d. none of the above

8. The wavelength is halved if

a. the frequency is halved

b. the frequency is doubled

c. the velocity is doubled

d. none of the above

9. What is the approximate reflection percentage from a fat-bone interface?

a. 1%

b. 25%

c. 50%

d. 100%

10. The angle of reflection at an interface is determined by

a. the angle of incidence

b. the angle of transmission

c. the frequency of the transducer

d. the velocity

11. A change in velocity as sound passes through an interface can cause

a. refraction

b. sidelobes

c. enhancement

d. none of the above

12. What affects the axial resolution?

a. spatial pulse length

b. wavelength

c. damping

d. all of the above

13. What affects the lateral resolution?

a. spatial pulse length

b. damping

c. focusing

d. all of the above

14. What is the effect of higher frequencies on attenuation and penetration?

a. less attenuation, less penetration

b. more attenuation, less penetration

c. more attenuation, more penetration

d. less attenuation, more penetration

15. What are the three categories of bioeffects?

a. heat, thermal, other

b. heat, thermal, cavitation

c. heat, cavitation, other

d. none of the above

16. Frequencies used for medical diagnostic ultrasound normally range from

a. 20 Hz to 20,000 Hz

b. 20 kHz to 20 MHz

c. 2 MHz to 15 MHz

d. 20 MHz to 40 MHz

17. The velocity of sound is greatest through

a. bone

b. fat

c. water

d. air

18. The value of 1% is related to a fat-muscle interface. This parameter is the

a. reflection coefficient

b. attenuation coefficient

c. refraction coefficient

d. transmission coefficient

19. Ultrasound includes only those frequencies above

a. 20 Hz

b. 20 kHz

c. 100 kHz

d. 1 MHz

20. Intensity can be measured in

a. milliwatts per centimeter

b. watts per meter

c. milliwatts

d. watts per square meter

21. What does not cause attenuation?

a. enhancement

b. absorption

c. scattering

d. reflection

22. If the velocities of the two materials that form an interface are not equal, and if the angle of incidence is not zero,

a. the reflected angle will not be the same as the incident angle

b. refraction may occur

c. the transmitted angle will always equal the incident angle

d. the quality factor will increase

23. Red blood cells

a. are specular reflectors

b. do not cause Rayleigh scattering

c. are nonspecular reflectors

d. do not reflect diagnostic ultrasound frequencies

24. The velocity of sound through a material is not affected by

a. stiffness

b. density

c. frequency

d. elasticity

25. The component that produces ultrasound energy is the

a. transducer

b. receiver

c. pulser

d. cathode ray tube

26. A perpendicular angle of incidence is

a. normal incidence

b. oblique incidence

c. critical incidence

d. an incident angle of 90 degrees

27. The velocity of sound through bone is in the range of

a. 300 to 1650 meters per second

b. 4000 to 5000 meters per second

c. 6000 to 8000 meters per second

d. 8000 to 10,000 meters per second

28. A nonspecular reflector will produce

a. transient cavitation

b. stable cavitation

c. 100% reflection coefficient

d. backscatter

29. What is one difference between audible and inaudible sound?

a. audible sound is above 20 kHz

b. inaudible sound waves are never longitudinal

c. audible sound is used for therapeutic applications

d. inaudible sound has a higher frequency

30. If the frequency is doubled,

a. the period will not change

b. the period will be doubled

c. the wavelength will be halved

d. the wavelength will be doubled

31. Extraneous energy components that are not in the primary direction of the ultrasound beam

a. will not affect the lateral resolution

b. will affect the axial resolution

c. are called sidelobes

d. can be eliminated by increasing the PRF

32. Which of the following does not affect axial (longitudinal) resolution?

a. focusing

b. frequency

c. spatial pulse length

d. damping

33. Lateral resolution is affected by all of the following except

a. frequency

b. beam width

c. focusing

d. bandwidth

34. Which transducer produces a sector image?

a. flat sequenced array

b. continuous wave Doppler probe

c. flat linear array

d. curved linear array

35. What is the shape of the image produced by a phased array transducer?

a. sector (pie-shaped)

b. linear (rectangular)

c. linear (pie-shaped)

d. linear (trapezoidal)

36. What is the shape of the image produced by a flat sequenced array?

a. sector (pie-shaped)

b. linear (rectangular)

c. linear (trapezoidal)

d. linear (pie-shaped)

37. What is the shape of the image produced by a convex array?

a. sector (rectangular)

b. sector (pie-shaped)

c. sector (trapezoidal)

d. linear (rectangular)

38. Which element arrangement is often used in mechanically steered transducers?

a. linear array

b. phased array

c. annular array

d. sequenced array

39. A decrease in the thickness of the piezoelectric element will result in

a. a decrease in the quality factor

b. an increase in the frequency of the transducer

c. an increase in the velocity of sound

d. a greater pulse duration

40. Lateral resolution is determined by

a. the angle of refraction

b. damping

c. spatial pulse length

d. beam width

41. Electronic focusing is possible with

a. single-element transducers

b. transducer arrays

c. two-element continuous wave Doppler probes

d. none of the above

42. Which of the following does not produce a sector image?

a. annual array

b. phased linear array

c. flat sequenced linear array

d. convex array

43. The Transmitter, Acoustic Power, or Energy Output control

a. affects the amplification of received echoes

b. varies the frequency of the transducer

c. affects the amount of energy entering a patient

d. varies the dynamic range

44. The duty factor in a pulse-echo system

a. is greater than the duty factor in a continuous wave Doppler system

b. is normally less than 1%

c. is typically 50%

d. is normally 100%

45. An ultrasound wave leaves the transducer, travels through tissue, and returns 10 microseconds later. What is the distance to the reflector?

a. 1.54 mm

b. 15.4 mm

c. 7.7 mm

d. 1540 meters

46. The beams from an annular array

a. have a rectangular-shaped cross section

b. are normally wider than beams from single-element transducers

c. cannot be electronically focused

d. cannot be electronically steered

47. If the real time frame rate is increased, the result will be

a. increased line density

b. decreased line density

c. a smoother image

d. none of the above

48. With phased array transducers, the transmitted sound beam is steered by

a. mechanically rotating three or more piezoelectric elements

b. increasing the PRF with each applied shock pulse

c. varying the delay of pulses to the transducer's elements

d. varying the frequency applied to the transducer's elements

49. Read Magnification is performed by

a. controlling the A to D converter

b. enlarging each pixel

c. placing a large magnifying glass over the TV screen

d. varying the Depth setting

50. What is the size of a typical image memory matrix?

a. 10×10

b. 10×256

c. 256×256

d. 512×512

51. How many horizontal scan lines are in a television frame?

a. 525

b. $262\frac{1}{2}$

c. 60

d. 30

52. The maximum number of displayed gray shades in an 8 bit system is

a. 8

b. 256

c. 64

d. 512

53. The number of TV fields per second is

a. 10

b. 30

c. 60

d. $262\frac{1}{2}$

54. A digital picture element is a

a. bit

b. voxel

c. pixel

d. none of the above

55. Which of the following is a "hard copy?"

a. floppy disk recording

b. multi-image film

c. videotape recording

d. optical disk recording

56. The output of the scan converter's D to A converter is fed to the

a. transducer

b. receiver

c. TV monitor

d. spectrum analyzer

57. What is the scan converter function that determines the assignment of echoes to predetermined gray scale levels?

a. post processing

b. pre processing

c. bit mapping

d. D to A conversion

58. What is the scan converter function that determines the CRT brightness assigned to the various gray scale levels?

a. log compression

b. A to D conversion

c. pre processing

d. post processing

59. A Doppler angle of 90 degrees results in

a. no Doppler shift

b. maximum Doppler shift

c. a shift to a higher frequency

d. a shift to a lower frequency

60. Aliasing will be present if the Doppler shift exceeds

a. the PRF

b. twice the PRF

c. one half the Nyquist limit

d. the Nyquist limit

61. The difference between red and blue hues in a color flow doppler image represents a difference in

a. reflection coefficient

b. reflector amplitude

c. flow intensity

d. flow direction

62. A high PRF, when using pulsed Doppler

a. increases the possibility of aliasing

b. increases the chances for depth ambiguity

c. eliminates the refraction artifact

d. decreases the chance of depth ambiguity

63. Which one of the following factors does not affect the frequency of the Doppler shift?

a. angle with which the probe is pointed at a vessel

b. velocity of blood in a vessel

c. the transmitted frequency

d. size of the Doppler probe

64. Continuous wave Doppler systems

a. are capable of detecting higher velocities than are gated Doppler systems

b. detect all movement in the path of the Doppler beam

c. both of the above

d. none of the above

65. Bioeffects have not been confirmed for SPTA intensities below

a. 100 mW per meter

b. 100 W per square cm

c. 100 mW per square cm

d. 10,000 mW per square cm

Chapter 2

INSTRUMENTATION

REVIEW QUESTIONS

1. Which of the following does not produce a sector image.

a. annular array

b. phased linear array

c. flat sequenced array

d. convex array

2. Increasing the Dynamic Range in a pulse-echo ultrasound system does not

a. ensure a wider range of displayed gray levels

b. decrease the amount of compression of the received signal

c. decrease the attenuation of sound in tissue

d. increase the ratio of the largest signal to the smallest signal that the system can handle

3. The component that generates ultrasound energy is the

a. transducer

b. receiver

c. pulser

d. cathode ray tube

4. The beams from an annular array

a. have a rectangular cross section

b. are normally wider than beams from single-element transducers

c. cannot be electronically focused

d. cannot be electronically steered

5. If the pulse repetition frequency is increased, the real time frame will have

a. a higher frame rate

b. a lower frame rate

c. more acoustic lines

d. fewer acoustic lines

6. Read Magnification is performed by

a. controlling the A to D converter

b. enlarging each pixel

c. placing a large magnifying glass over the TV screen

d. varying the depth setting

7. What is the size of a typical image memory matrix?

a. 10×10

b. 10×256

c. 256×256

d. 512×512

8. How many horizontal scan lines are contained in a television frame?

a. 525

b. $262\frac{1}{2}$

c. 60

d. 30

9. The maximum number of displayed gray shades in an 8-bit system is

a. 8

b. 256

c. 64

d. 512

10. The output of the scan converter is fed to the

a. transducer

b. receiver

c. TV monitor

d. spectrum analyzer

11. What is the scan converter function that determines the assignment of echoes to predetermined gray scale levels?

a. postprocessing

b. preprocessing

c. bit mapping

d. D to A conversion

12. Which of the following performs digital storage of echo-signal information?

a. scan converter

b. TV monitor

c. receiver

d. A to D converter

13. An advantage of continuous wave Doppler over pulsed Doppler is

a. a lower Nyquist limit

b. a lower PRF

c. a wider range of shift frequencies

d. spectral analysis is not required

14. Aliasing will be present if the Doppler shift exceeds

a. the PRF

b. twice the PRF

c. one half the Nyquist limit

d. the Nyquist limit

15. A low PRF, when using pulse Doppler

a. detects a wider range of shift frequencies than continuous wave Doppler

b. will not result in aliasing if the Doppler shift is higher than the PRF

c. may result in aliasing when high velocity flow is present

d. will not result in aliasing if the Doppler shift is equal to the PRF

Chapter 3

BODY SYSTEMS

REVIEW QUESTIONS

1. All of the following are tasks performed by bones except

  a. protection

  b. support

  c. blood cell formation

  d. hormone release

2. Voluntary muscles include all of the following except

  a. biceps

  b. cardiac

  c. triceps

  d. quadriceps

3. All of the following act as storage areas except

  a. spleen

  b. liver

  c. bone

  d. brain

4. Which of the following organs has two sets of capillary beds?

  a. liver

  b. kidneys

  c. pancreas

  d. spleen

5. Which organ allows free mixing of oxygenated and deoxygenated blood within sinusoids?

  a. liver

  b. kidneys

  c. pancreas

  d. spleen

6. Which organ is dependent on subatmospheric pressures in order to perform properly?

  a. liver

  b. skin

  c. kidneys

  d. lungs

7. Which glands release a watery substance that assists in temperature control?

  a. ovaries

  b. testicles

  c. pancreas

  d. sweat glands

  e. sebaceous glands

8. Which of the following does not excrete urea?

  a. lungs

  b. kidneys

  c. skin

9. The ovum is released on approximately the _____ day of the menstrual cycle.

  a. fifth

  b. tenth

  c. fourteenth

  d. twenty-first

10. Which region of the brain is responsible for detecting changes in blood chemistry (receptors)?

  a. pituitary

  b. hypothalamus

  c. vermis

  d. cortical mantle

9

11. Which system requires a pump in order to circulate fluids?

a. arterial flow

b. venous flow

c. lymphatic flow

12. The structures within the GI tract that allow for expansion and contraction of the digestive wall, similar to an accordion, are

a. villi

b. rugae

c. tunica media

13. Which cavity contains the brain?

a. abdominopelvic

b. thoracic

c. spinal

d. cranial

14. Venous and lymphatic flow is primarily accomplished via

a. subatmospheric pressure

b. cardiac systolic contractions

c. muscle contraction

d. gravity

15. Which system is primarily responsible for removing excess fluids and preventing edema?

a. lymphatic

b. circulatory

c. digestive

d. endocrine

16. The pleural sac is associated with the

a. heart

b. lungs

c. kidneys

d. spleen

17. Fertilization usually occurs in the

a. uterus

b. ovary

c. fallopian tube

d. cervix

18. All of the following areas have capillary blood flow except

a. hypodermis

b. dermis

c. epidermis

19. Which hormone causes a decrease in blood sugar levels?

a. epinephrine

b. norepinephrine

c. glucagon

d. insulin

20. Which organ is not part of the excretory system?

a. skin

b. kidney

c. adrenal gland

d. lung

Identify the structures indicated in the following illustrations. These figures duplicate those found in **ULTRASONOGRAPHY: Introduction to Normal Structure and Functional Anatomy**. Refer to the textbook if you need help.

1 _____

2 _____

3 _____

4 _____

5 _____

6 _____

7 _____

8 _____

9 _____

10 _____

11 _____

12 _____

13 _____

14 _____

15 _____

16 _____

17 _____

18 _____

19 _____

20 _____

21 _____

22 _____

23 _____

24 _____

25 _____

26 _____

27 _____

Veins of the circulatory system.

28 _____

29 _____

30 _____

31 _____

Arteries

42
41
40
39
38
37
36
35
34
33
32
31
30
29
28
27
26
25
24
23
22
21
20
19
18
17
16

1
2
3
4
5
6

to vein

15
14

venule

13
12
11
10
9
8
7

A capillary bed

Arteries of the circulatory system.

1 _____

2 _____

3 _____

4 _____

5 _____

6 _____

7 _____

8 _____

9 _____

10 _____

11 _____

12 _____

13 _____

14 _____

15 _____

16 _____

17 _____

18 _____

19 _____

20 _____

21 _____

22 _____

23 _____

24 _____

25 _____

26 _____

27 _____

28 _____

29 _____

30 _____

31 _____

32 _____

33 _____

34 _____

35 _____

36 _____

37 _____

38 _____

39 _____

40 _____

41 _____

42 _____

1 _____

2 _____

3 _____

4 _____

5 _____

6 _____

7 _____

8 _____

9 _____

10 _____

11 _____

12 _____

13 _____

14 _____

15 _____

16 _____

17 _____

18 _____

19 _____

20 _____

21 _____

22 _____

23 _____

24 _____

25 _____

26 _____

27 _____

28 _____

29 _____

30 _____

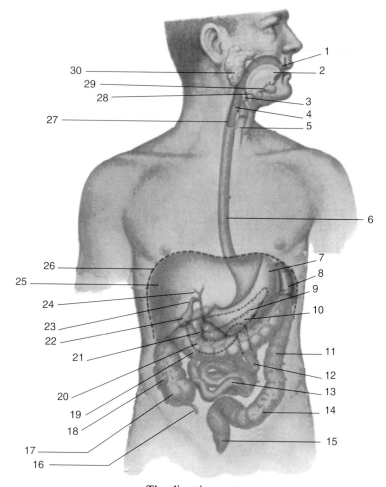

The digestive system.

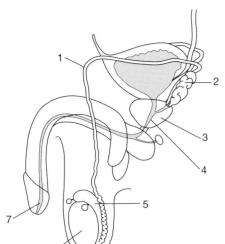

Male reproductive system.

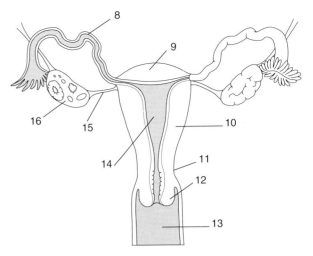

Female reproductive system.

1 _____	9 _____
2 _____	10 _____
3 _____	11 _____
4 _____	12 _____
5 _____	13 _____
6 _____	14 _____
7 _____	15 _____
8 _____	16 _____

1 _____
2 _____
3 _____
4 _____
5 _____
6 _____
7 _____
8 _____
9 _____
10 _____
11 _____
12 _____
13 _____

inner ear:

The ear; the eye.

14 _____
15 _____
16 _____
17 _____

1 _____

2 _____

3 _____

4 _____

5 _____

6 _____

7 _____

8 _____

9 _____

10 _____

11 _____

12 _____

13 _____

14 _____

Middle and inner ear.

15 _____

16 _____

17 _____

18 _____

19 _____

1 _____

2 _____

3 _____

4 _____

5 _____

6 _____

7 _____

8 _____

9 _____

10 _____

11 _____

12 _____

13 _____

14 _____

15 _____

16 _____

Horizontal section of the eye.

17 _____

18 _____

19 _____

20 _____

21 _____

22 _____

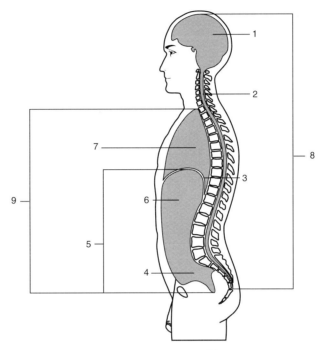

Figure 3–1. Body cavities.

1 _____   6 _____

2 _____   7 _____

3 _____   8 _____

4 _____   9 _____

5 _____

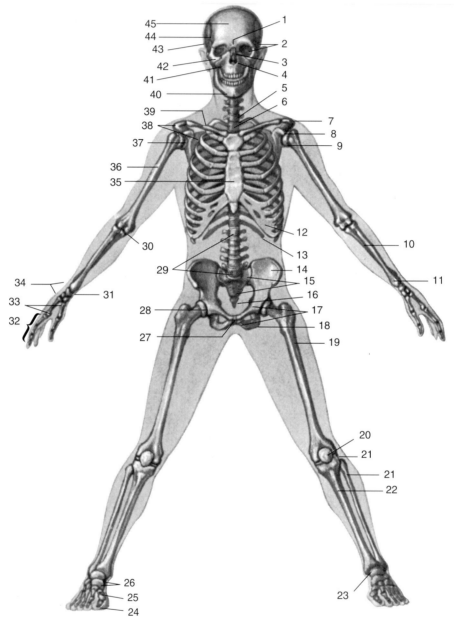

Figure 3-2. Skeletal bones.

1 _____

2 _____

3 _____

4 _____

5 _____

6 _____

7 _____

8 _____

9 _____

10 _____

11 _____

12 _____

13 _____

14 _____

15 _____

16 _____

17 _____

18 _____

19 _____

20 _____

21 _____

22 _____

23 _____

24 _____

25 _____

26 _____

27 _____

28 _____

29 _____

30 _____

31 _____

32 _____

33 _____

34 _____

35 _____

36 _____

37 _____

38 _____

39 _____

40 _____

41 _____

42 _____

43 _____

44 _____

45 _____

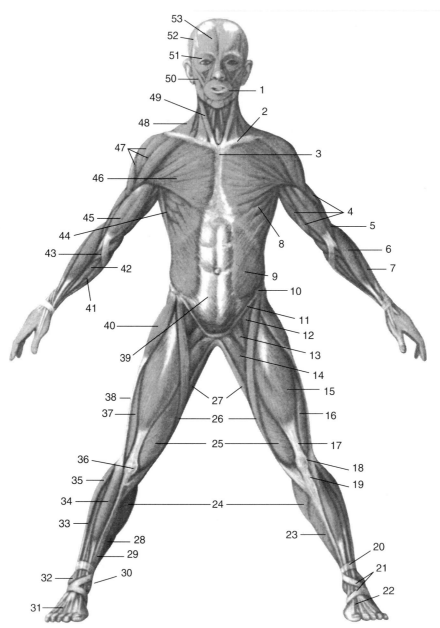

Figure 3–2. *Continued.* Skeletal muscles.

1 _____

2 _____

3 _____

4 _____

5 _____

6 _____

7 _____

8 _____

9 _____

10 _____

11 _____

12 _____

13 _____

14 _____

15 _____

16 _____

17 _____

18 _____

19 _____

20 _____

21 _____

22 _____

23 _____

24 _____

25 _____

26 _____

27 _____

28 _____

29 _____

30 _____

31 _____

32 _____

33 _____

34 _____

35 _____

36 _____

37 _____

38 _____

39 _____

40 _____

41 _____

42 _____

43 _____

44 _____

45 _____

46 _____

47 _____

48 _____

49 _____

50 _____

51 _____

52 _____

53 _____

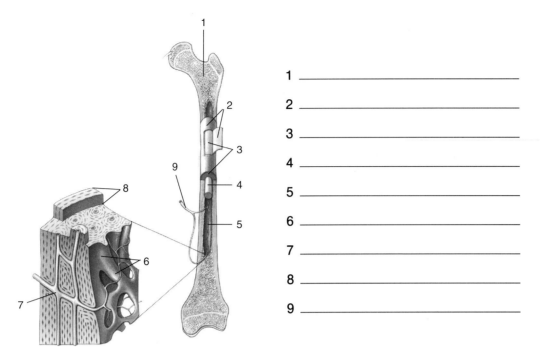

Figure 3-3.   Bone composition.

1 _____

2 _____

3 _____

4 _____

5 _____

6 _____

7 _____

8 _____

9 _____

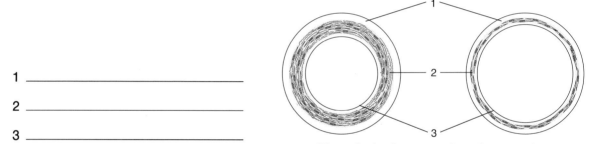

1 _____

2 _____

3 _____

Figure 3-4.   Structure of arteries and veins.

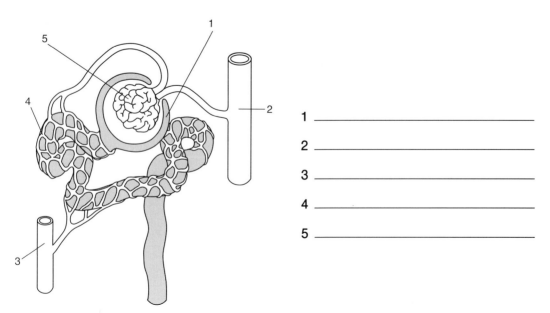

Figure 3-5.   The two capillary beds of the kidney.

1 _____

2 _____

3 _____

4 _____

5 _____

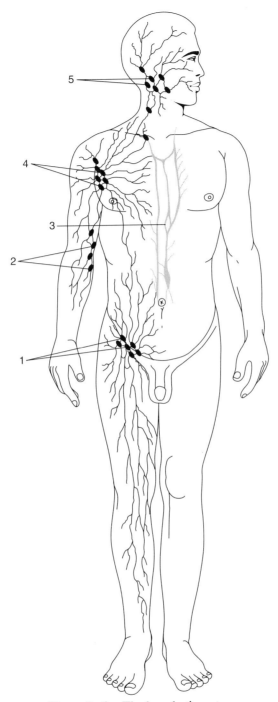

Figure 3-6. The lymphatic system.

1 _____

2 _____

3 _____

4 _____

5 _____

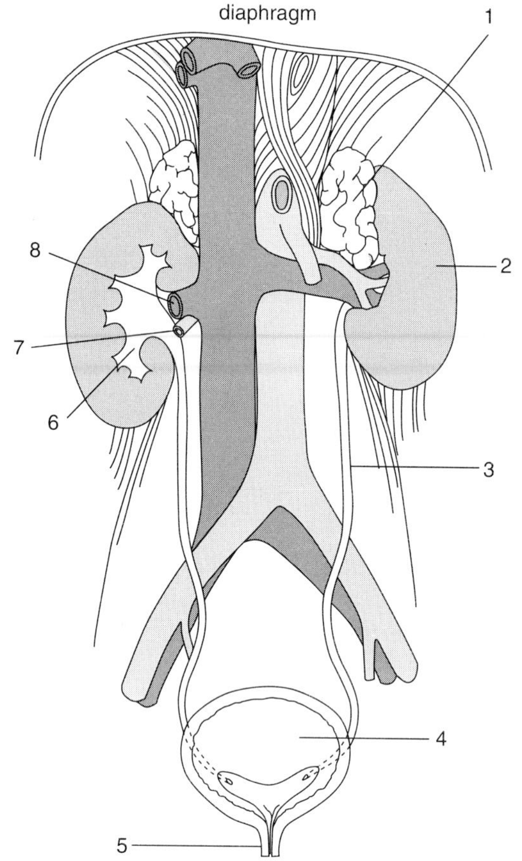

Figure 3-7. The urinary system.

1 _____
2 _____
3 _____
4 _____
5 _____
6 _____
7 _____
8 _____

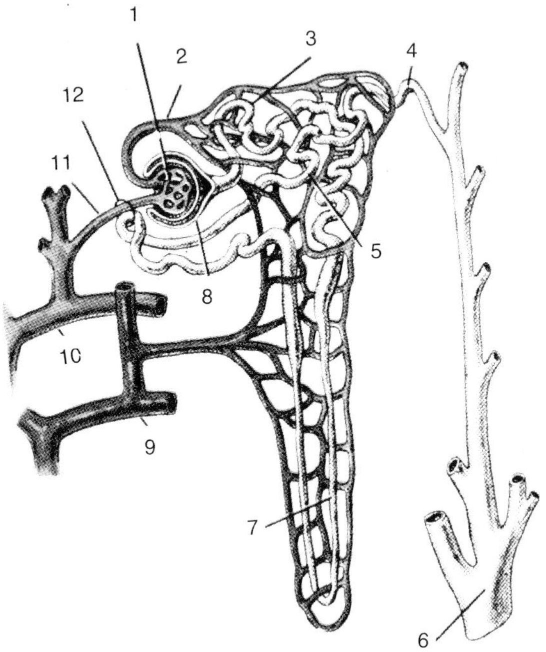

Figure 3-8. A nephron and surrounding capillaries. (From Guyton, A.C.: Textbook of Medical Physiology, 6th ed. Philadelphia, W.B. Saunders Company, 1981).

1 _____
2 _____
3 _____
4 _____
5 _____
6 _____
7 _____
8 _____
9 _____

10 _____
11 _____
12 _____

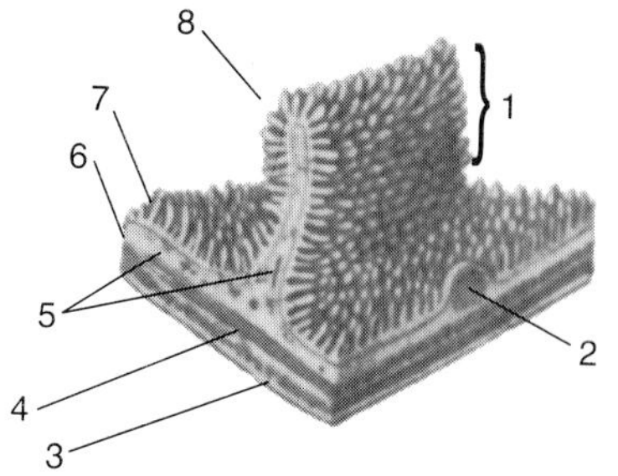

Figure 3-9. Section of small intestine wall.

1 _____
2 _____
3 _____
4 _____
5 _____
6 _____
7 _____
8 _____

1 _____

2 _____

3 _____

4 _____

5 _____

6 _____

7 _____

8 _____

9 _____

10 _____

11 _____

12 _____

13 _____

14 _____

15 _____

16 _____

17 _____

18 _____

19 _____

20 _____

21 _____

22 _____

23 _____

24 _____

25 _____

26 _____

27 _____

28 _____

29 _____

30 _____

31 _____

32 _____

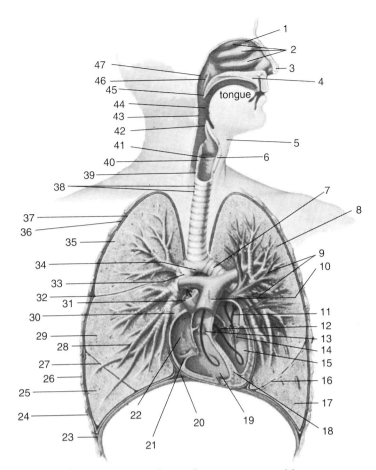

Figure 3–10A. The respiratory system and heart.

33 _____

34 _____

35 _____

36 _____

37 _____

38 _____

39 _____

40 _____

41 _____

42 _____

43 _____

44 _____

45 _____

46 _____

47 _____

1 _____

2 _____

3 _____

4 _____

5 _____

6 _____

7 _____

8 _____

9 _____

10 _____

11 _____

12 _____

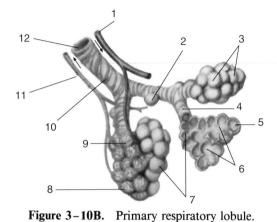

Figure 3–10B. Primary respiratory lobule.

1 _____

2 _____

3 _____

4 _____

5 _____

6 _____

7 _____

8 _____

9 _____

10 _____

11 _____

12 _____

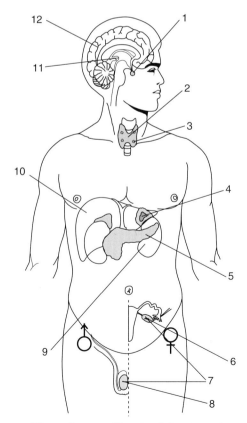

Figure 3–11. Glands of the endocrine system.

Chapter 4

ANATOMY LAYERING AND SECTIONAL ANATOMY

REVIEW QUESTIONS

1. Which structure is *not* intraperitoneal?

a. gallbladder

b. pancreas

c. liver

d. spleen

2. Which structure is *not* retroperitoneal?

a. gallbladder

b. pancreas

c. urinary bladder

d. aorta

3. Which structure does *not* lie in a vertical position within the body?

a. abdominal aorta

b. superior mesenteric vein

c. left renal vein

d. superior mesenteric artery

4. Which structure does *not* lie transversely within the body?

a. left renal vein

b. left renal artery

c. portal vein

d. right renal vein

5. Which anatomic area is *not* seen on a sagittal section?

a. posterior

b. inferior

c. anterior

d. medial

6. Which anatomic area is *not* seen on a coronal section?

a. medial

b. lateral

c. anterior

d. superior

7. Which anatomic area is *not* seen on a transverse section?

a. superior

b. right lateral

c. anterior

d. medial

8. The scanning planes used in sonography are the same as anatomic body planes, but their interpretations are dependent upon:

a. the size of the transducer

b. the shape of the transducer and how it is held

c. body habitus

d. the location of the transducer and the sound wave approach.

9. The single difference between structures seen on an ultrasound image section and a cadaver section is:

a. size

b. sonographic appearance

c. adjacent relationships

d. shape

10. Which term is *not* used to describe sonographic appearance?

a. isosonic

b. annular array

c. anechoic

d. hypoechoic

11. Using the figure below: the pancreas is located _____ to the splenic artery.

a. inferior

b. anterior

c. posterior

d. superior

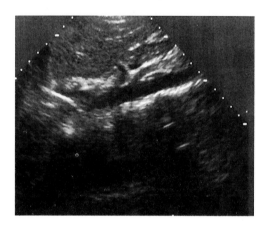
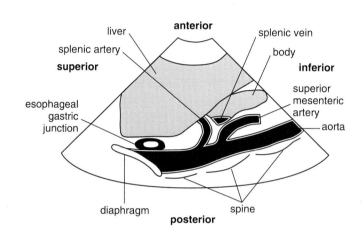

12. Using the figure below: the psoas muscle is located _____ to the aorta.

a. superior

b. lateral

c. medial

d. inferior

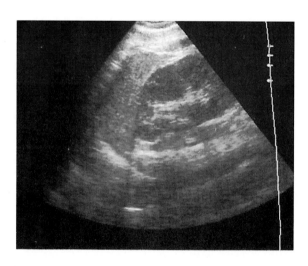
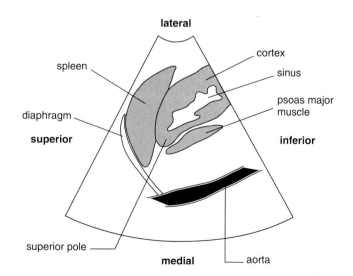

13. Using the figure below: the left renal vein is located _____ to the superior mesenteric artery.

a. anterior

b. posterior

c. left lateral

d. right lateral

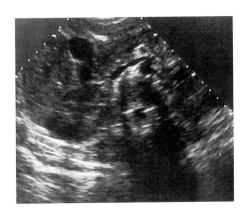

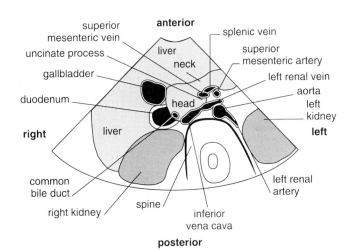

14. Using the figure below: the superior mesenteric vein is located _____ to the superior mesenteric artery.

a. left lateral

b. posterior

c. right lateral

d. anterior

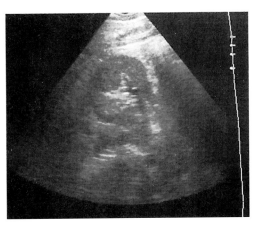

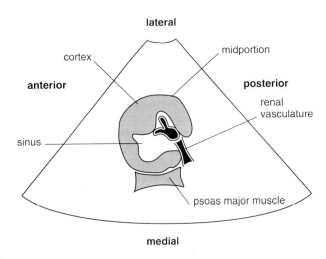

15. Using the figure above: the superior mesenteric vein runs between the _____ and _____ .

a. splenic vein and inferior vena cava

b. splenic vein and aorta

c. pancreas neck and uncinate process

d. pancreas head and inferior vena cava

Identify the structures indicated in the following illustrations. These figures duplicate those found in **ULTRASONOGRAPHY: Introduction to Normal Structure and Functional Anatomy**. Refer to the textbook if you need help.

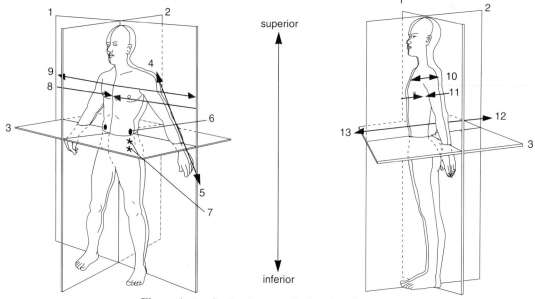

Figure 4–1. Body planes and directional terms.

1 _____   8 _____

2 _____   9 _____

3 _____   10 _____

4 _____   11 _____

5 _____   12 _____

6 _____   13 _____

7 _____

---

1 _____   12 _____

2 _____   13 _____

3 _____   14 _____

4 _____   15 _____

5 _____   16 _____

6 _____   17 _____

7 _____   18 _____

8 _____   19 _____

9 _____   20 _____

10 _____   21 _____

11 _____

REGIONAL DIVISIONS OF THE ABDOMEN

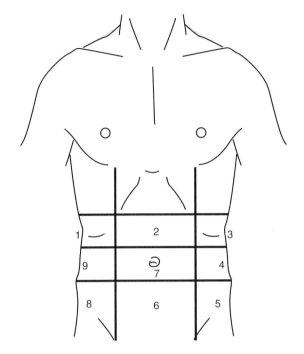

QUADRANT DIVISIONS OF THE ABDOMEN

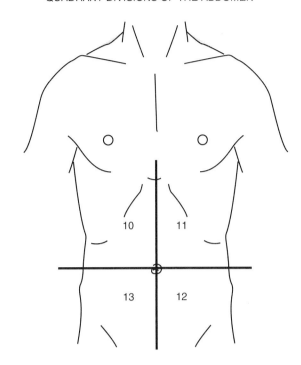

SURFACE LANDMARKS OF THE ABDOMINAL WALL

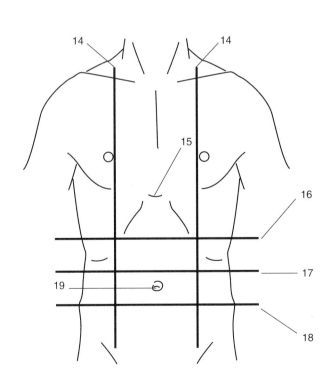

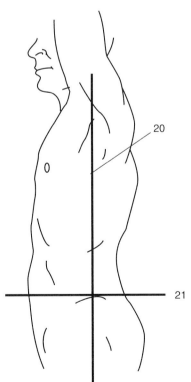

Figure 4–2.

THE LAYERS OF THE ABDOMEN

A. POSTERIOR MUSCLES

right   left

1 _____

2 _____

3 _____

4 _____

5 _____

1 _____

2 _____

3 _____

4 _____

5 _____

6 _____

7 _____

8 _____

9 _____

10 _____

B. KIDNEYS AND ADRENAL GLANDS

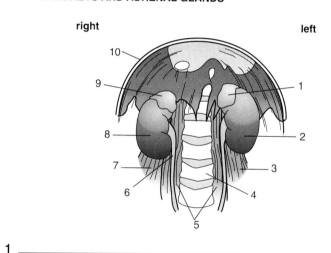

right   left

1 _____

2 _____

3 _____

4 _____

5 _____

6 _____

7 _____

8 _____

9 _____

10 _____

11 _____

12 _____

13 _____

C. VENA CAVA

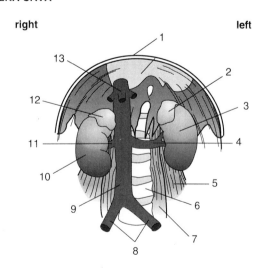

right   left

Figure 4–3.

1 _____

2 _____

3 _____

4 _____

5 _____

6 _____

7 _____

8 _____

9 _____

10 _____

11 _____

12 _____

13 _____

14 _____

15 _____

16 _____

17 _____

D. AORTA

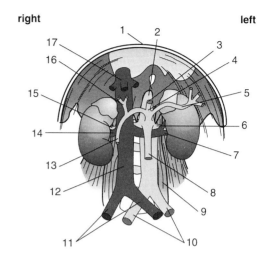

1 _____

2 _____

3 _____

4 _____

5 _____

6 _____

7 _____

8 _____

9 _____

10 _____

11 _____

12 _____

13 _____

14 _____

15 _____

16 _____

17 _____

18 _____

E. PORTAL VENOUS SYSTEM

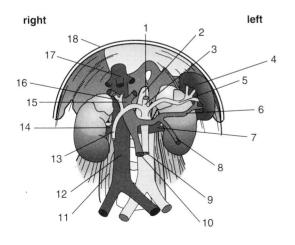

Figure 4–3. *Continued*

F. PANCREAS

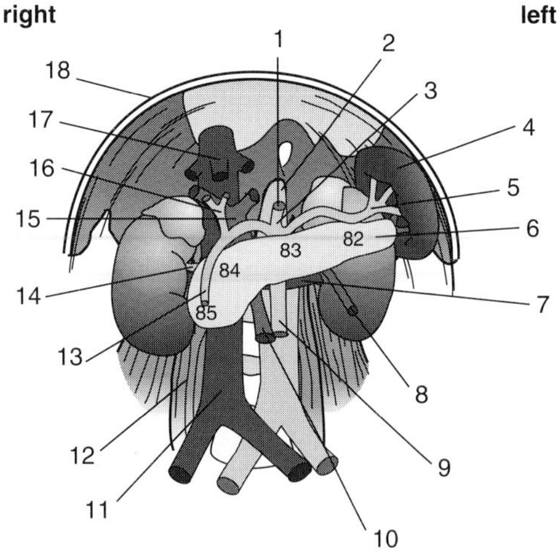

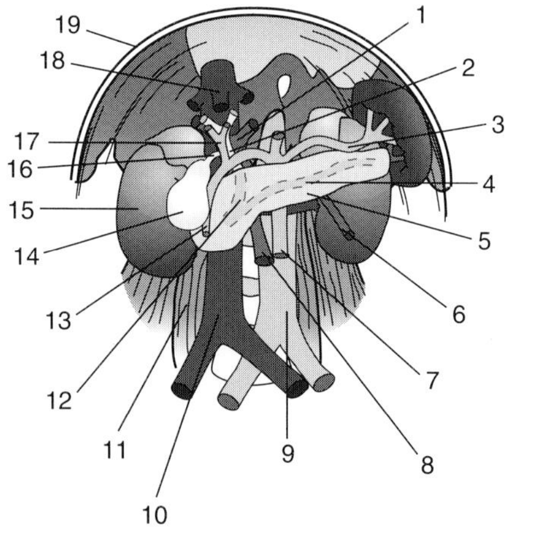

right   left

1 _____

2 _____

3 _____

4 _____

5 _____

6 _____

7 _____

8 _____

9 _____

10 _____

11 _____

12 _____

13 _____

14 _____

15 _____

16 _____

17 _____

18 _____

1 _____

2 _____

3 _____

4 _____

5 _____

6 _____

7 _____

8 _____

9 _____

10 _____

11 _____

12 _____

13 _____

14 _____

15 _____

G. GALLBLADDER AND BILIARY TRACT

right   left

16 _____

17 _____

18 _____

19 _____

Figure 4–3. *Continued*

H. GASTROINTESTINAL TRACT

right   left

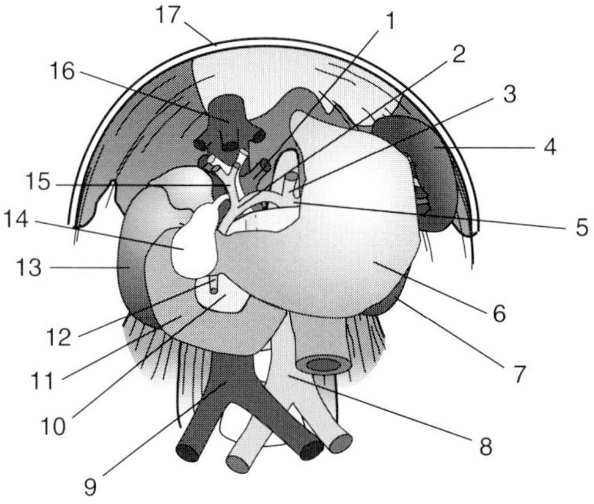

1 _____

2 _____

3 _____

4 _____

1 _____

2 _____

3 _____

4 _____

5 _____

6 _____

7 _____

8 _____

9 _____

J. ANTERIOR MUSCLES

right   left

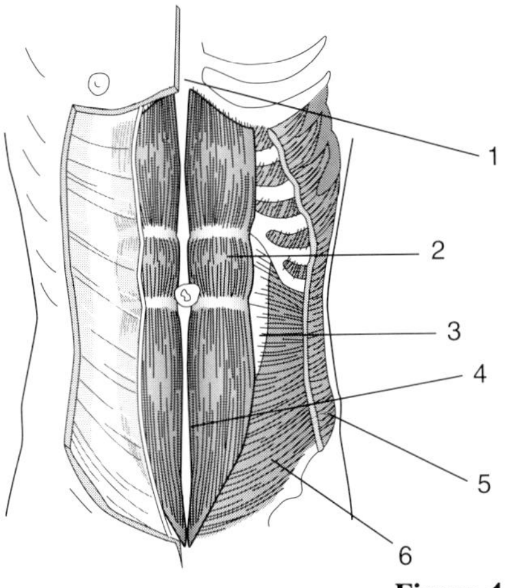

5 _____

6 _____

7 _____

8 _____

9 _____

10 _____

11 _____

12 _____

13 _____

14 _____

15 _____

16 _____

17 _____

I. LIVER

right   left

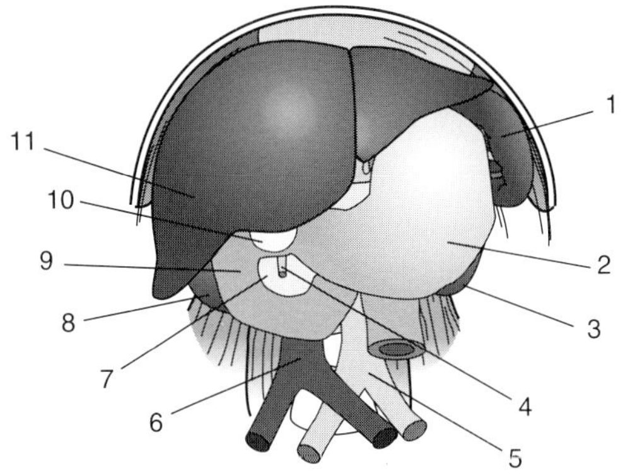

10 _____

11 _____

1 _____

2 _____

3 _____

4 _____

5 _____

6 _____

Figure 4–3. *Continued*

35

THE LAYERS OF THE PELVIS

A. POSTERIOR MUSCLES/TRUE PELVIS

right   left

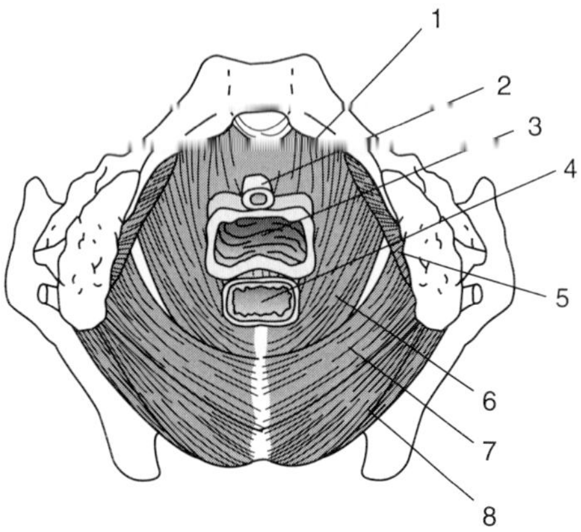

1 _____

2 _____

3 _____

4 _____

5 _____

6 _____

7 _____

8 _____

B. POSTERIOR MUSCLES/FALSE PELVIS

right   left

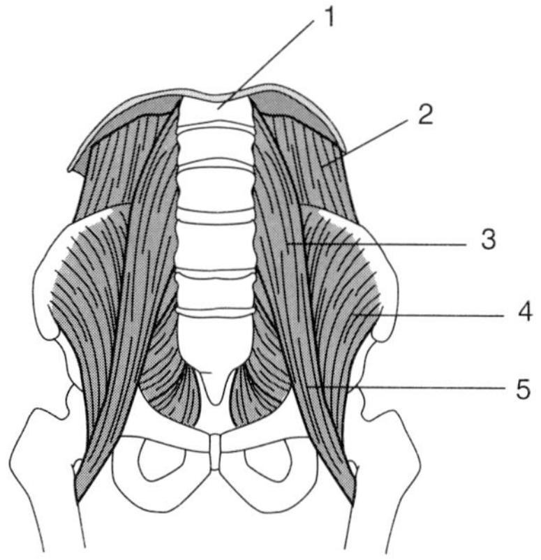

1 _____

2 _____

3 _____

4 _____

5 _____

C. RECTUM/COLON

right   left

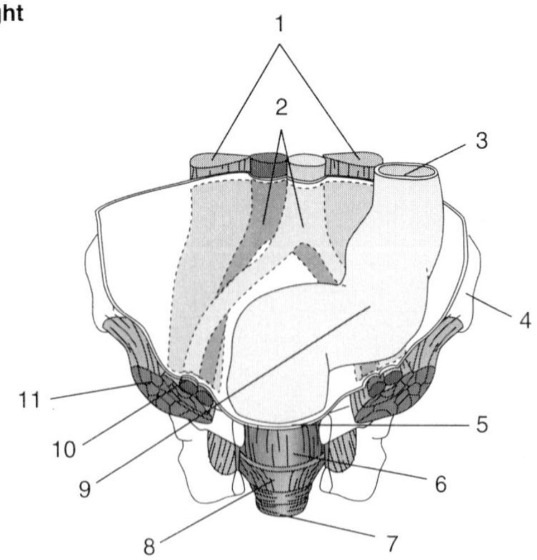

1 _____

2 _____

3 _____

4 _____

5 _____

6 _____

7 _____

8 _____

9 _____

10 _____

11 _____

Figure 4-4.

1 ______

2 ______

3 ______

4 ______

5 ______

6 ______

7 ______

8 ______

9 ______

10 ______

D. UTERUS/BLADDER

right
left
1
2
3
4
5
6
7
8
9
10

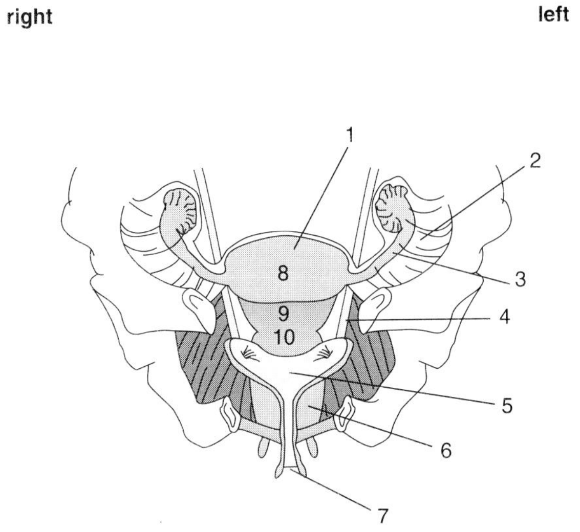

E. PROSTATE GLAND/BLADDER

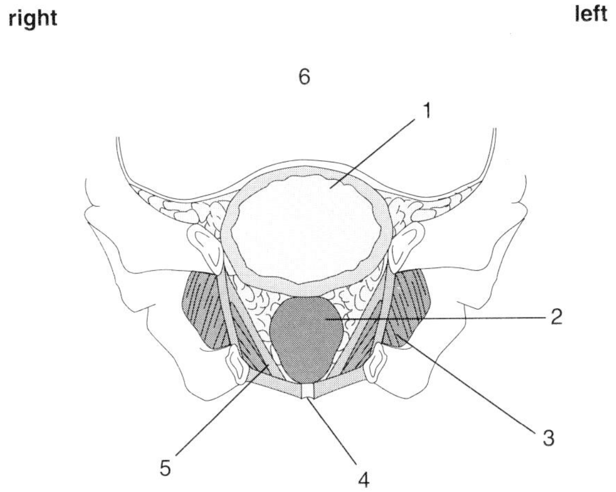

right
left
6
1
2
3
4
5

1 ______

2 ______

3 ______

4 ______

5 ______

6 ______

1 ______

2 ______

3 ______

F. ANTERIOR MUSCLE

right
left
1
2
3

Figure 4–4. *Continued*

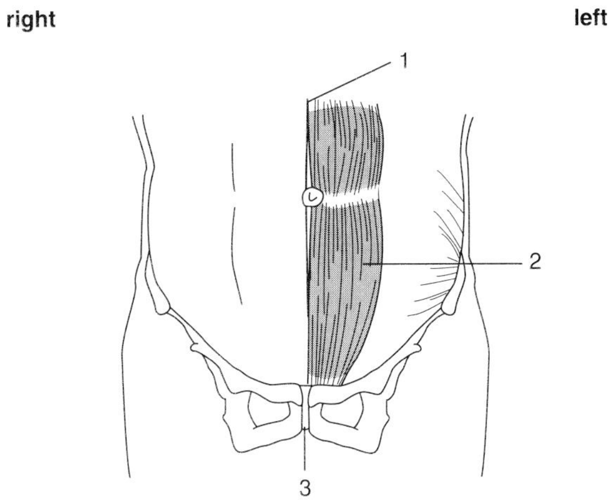

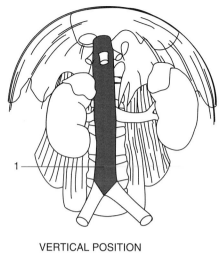

VERTICAL POSITION

1 _____

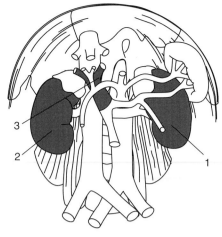

VERTICAL OBLIQUE POSITION

1 _____

2 _____

3 _____

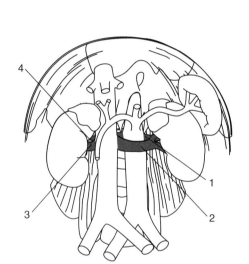

TRANSVERSE POSITION

1 _____

2 _____

3 _____

4 _____

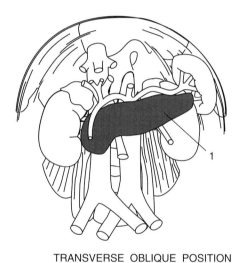

TRANSVERSE OBLIQUE POSITION

1 _____

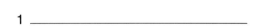

1 _____

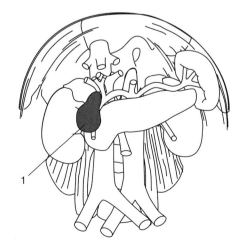

VARIABLE POSITION

Figure 4–5.

A. ANTERIOR APPROACH/SAGITTAL PLANE

note: transducer always
touches the skin surface

1 _____

2 _____

3 _____

4 _____

B. POSTERIOR APPROACH/SAGITTAL PLANE

1 _____

2 _____

3 _____

4 _____

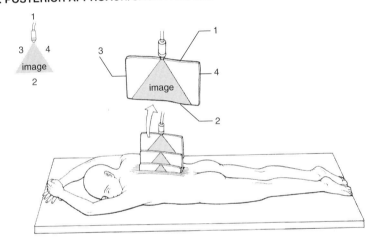

C. ANTERIOR APPROACH/TRANSVERSE PLANE

1 _____

2 _____

3 _____

4 _____

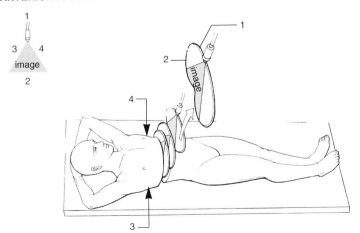

Figure 4–6.

D. POSTERIOR APPROACH/TRANSVERSE PLANE

1 _____

2 _____

3 _____

4 _____

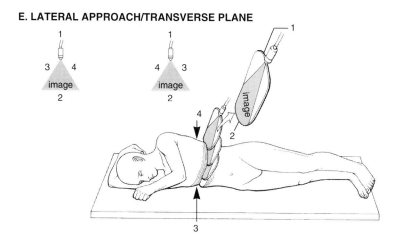

E. LATERAL APPROACH/TRANSVERSE PLANE

1 _____

2 _____

3 _____

4 _____

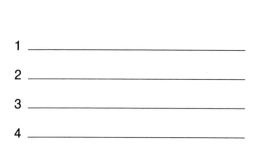

F. LATERAL APPROACH/CORONAL PLANE

1 _____

2 _____

3 _____

4 _____

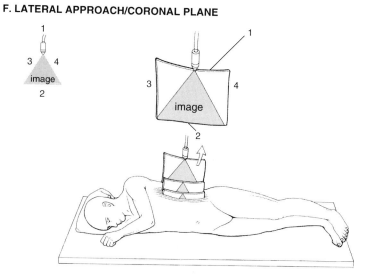

Figure 4–6. *Continued*

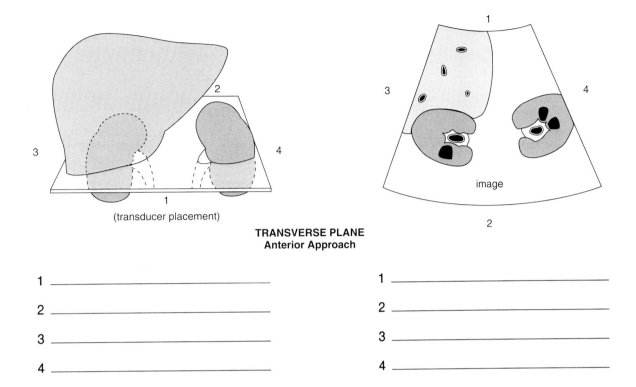

TRANSVERSE PLANE
Anterior Approach

(transducer placement)

1 _____

2 _____

3 _____

4 _____

1 _____

2 _____

3 _____

4 _____

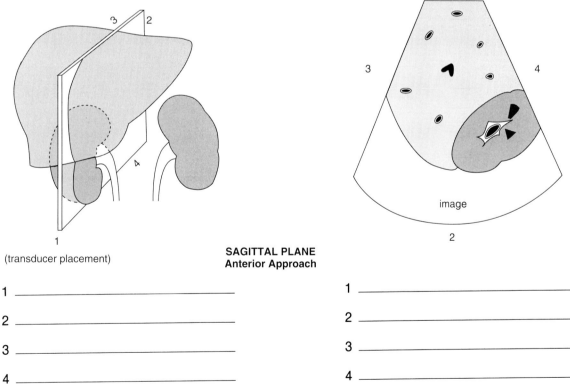

SAGITTAL PLANE
Anterior Approach

(transducer placement)

1 _____

2 _____

3 _____

4 _____

1 _____

2 _____

3 _____

4 _____

Figure 4–7.

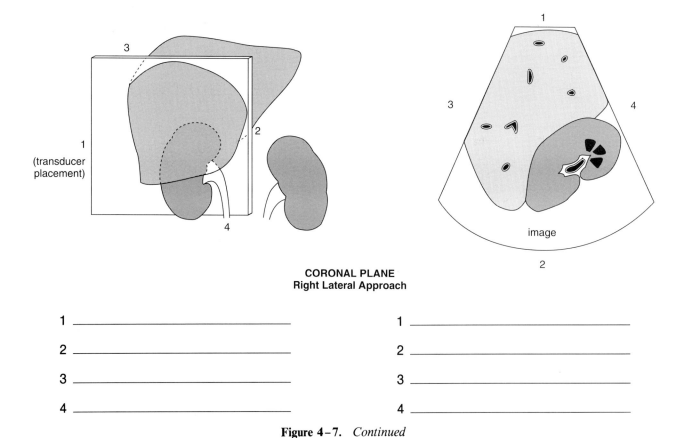

CORONAL PLANE
Right Lateral Approach

1 _____   1 _____

2 _____   2 _____

3 _____   3 _____

4 _____   4 _____

Figure 4–7. *Continued*

ENDOVAGINAL IMAGING

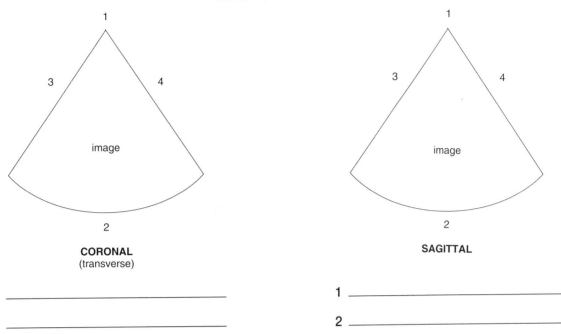

CORONAL
(transverse)

1 _____

2 _____

3 _____

4 _____

SAGITTAL

1 _____

2 _____

3 _____

4 _____

ENDORECTAL IMAGING

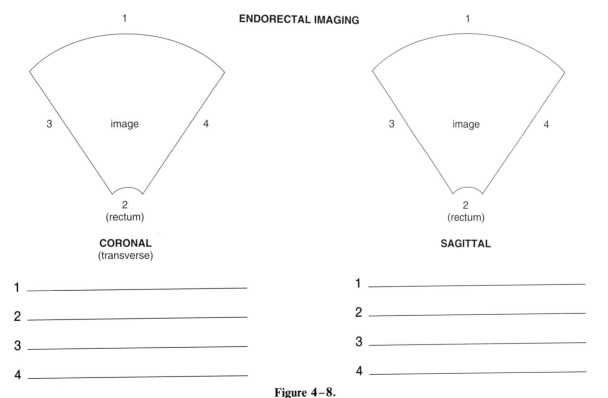

CORONAL
(transverse)

1 _____

2 _____

3 _____

4 _____

SAGITTAL

1 _____

2 _____

3 _____

4 _____

Figure 4–8.

NEUROSONOGRAPHY IMAGING
(Brain Imaging)

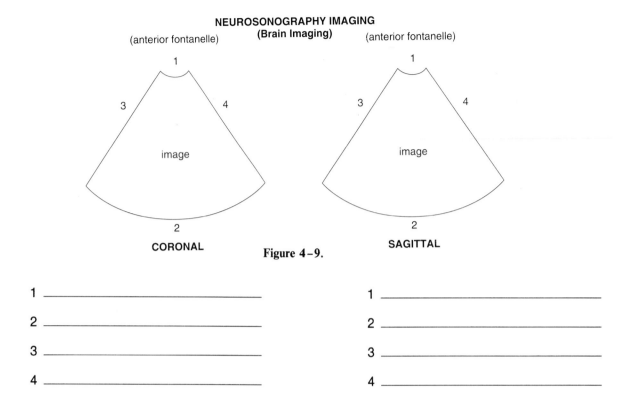

Figure 4-9.

1 _____
2 _____
3 _____
4 _____

1 _____
2 _____
3 _____
4 _____

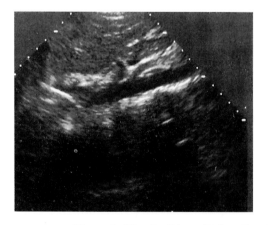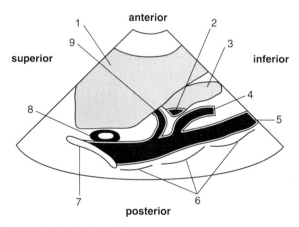

Figure 4-10. In this sagittal section the area of interest is the body of the pancreas.

1 _____
2 _____
3 _____
4 _____
5 _____

6 _____
7 _____
8 _____
9 _____

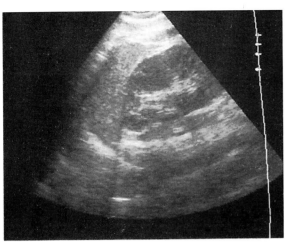
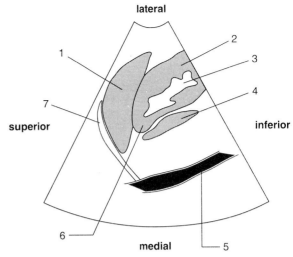

Figure 4–11. In this coronal section the area of interest is the superior pole of the left kidney.

1 _____   5 _____

2 _____   6 _____

3 _____   7 _____

4 _____

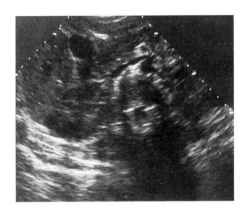
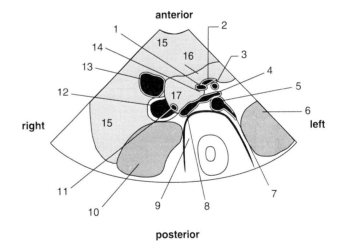

Figure 4–12. In this transverse section the area of interest is the head of the pancreas.

1 _____   10 _____

2 _____   11 _____

3 _____   12 _____

4 _____   13 _____

5 _____   14 _____

6 _____   15 _____

7 _____   16 _____

8 _____   17 _____

9 _____

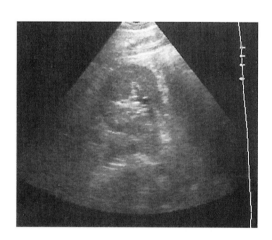 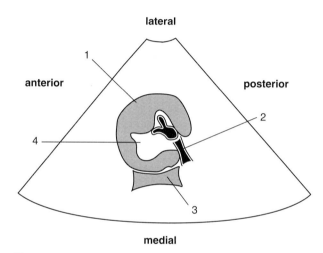

Figure 4–13. In this transverse section the area of interest is the midportion of the left kidney.

1 _____

2 _____

3 _____

4 _____

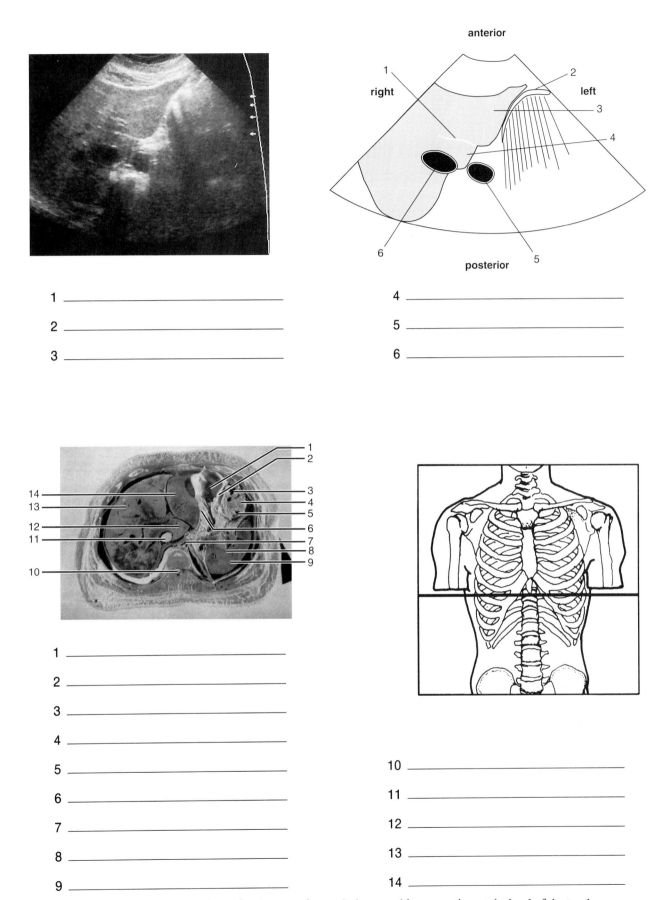

1 _____

2 _____

3 _____

4 _____

5 _____

6 _____

1 _____

2 _____

3 _____

4 _____

5 _____

6 _____

7 _____

8 _____

9 _____

10 _____

11 _____

12 _____

13 _____

14 _____

Figure 4–14. Comparison of cadaver section and ultrasound image section at the level of the tenth thoracic vertebrae.

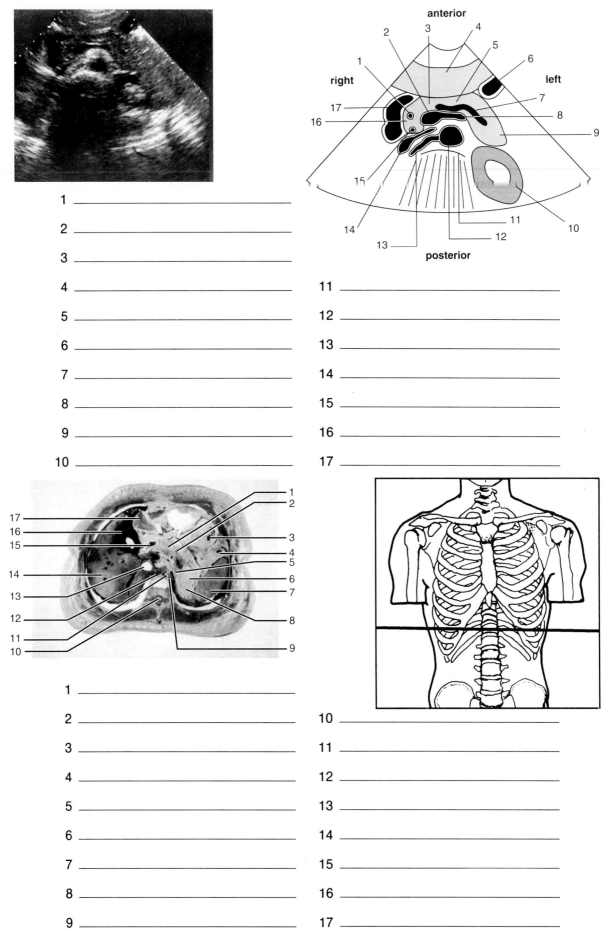

1 _____

2 _____

3 _____

4 _____   11 _____

5 _____   12 _____

6 _____   13 _____

7 _____   14 _____

8 _____   15 _____

9 _____   16 _____

10 _____   17 _____

1 _____

2 _____

3 _____

4 _____   10 _____

5 _____   11 _____

6 _____   12 _____

7 _____   13 _____

8 _____   14 _____

9 _____   15 _____

                              16 _____

                              17 _____

Figure 4–14. *Continued.* Comparison of cadaver section and ultrasound image section at the level of the twelfth thoracic vertebrae.

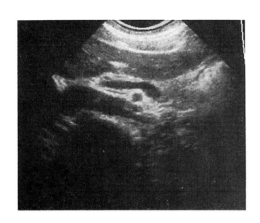

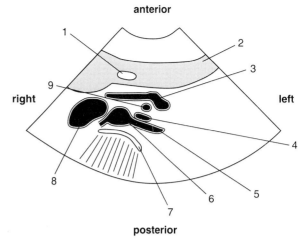

1 _____

2 _____

3 _____

4 _____

5 _____

6 _____

7 _____

8 _____

9 _____

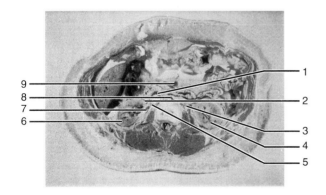

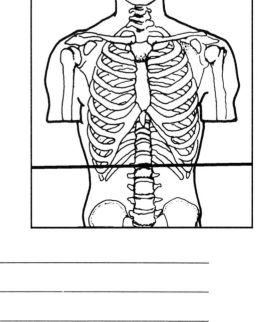

1 _____

2 _____

3 _____

4 _____

5 _____

6 _____

7 _____

8 _____

9 _____

Figure 4–14. *Continued.* Comparison of cadaver section and ultrasound image section at the level of the second lumbar vertebra.

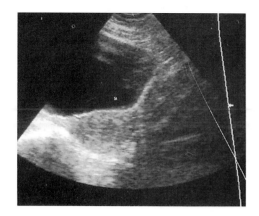

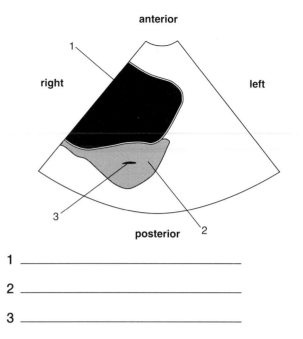

1 _____

2 _____

3 _____

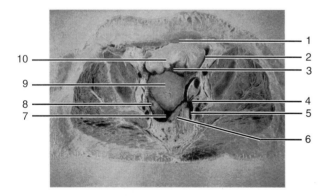

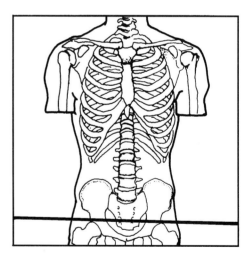

1 _____   6 _____

2 _____   7 _____

3 _____   8 _____

4 _____   9 _____

5 _____   10 _____

Figure 4–14. *Continued.* Comparison of cadaver section and ultrasound image section at the level of the fifth vertebra of the sacrum.

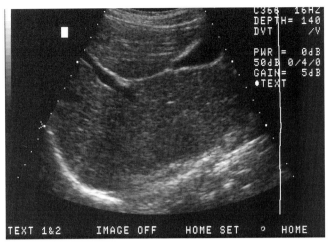 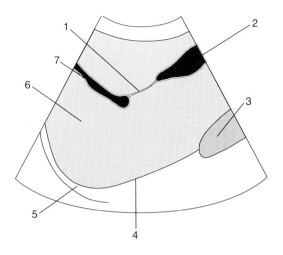

Figure 4–15. Right upper quadrant sagittal section.

1 _____   5 _____

2 _____   6 _____

3 _____   7 _____

4 _____

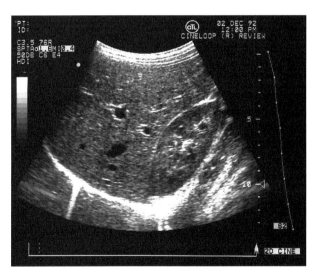 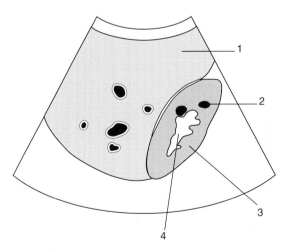

Figure 4–16. Right upper quadrant sagittal section.

1 _____   3 _____

2 _____   4 _____

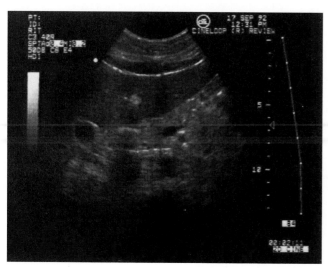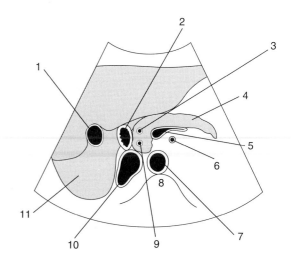

Figure 4–17. Epigastric transverse section.

1 _____   7 _____

2 _____   8 _____

3 _____   9 _____

4 _____   10 _____

5 _____   11 _____

6 _____

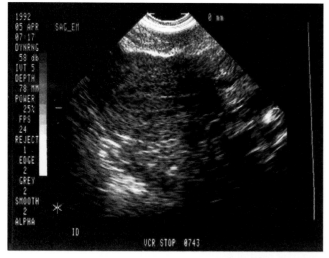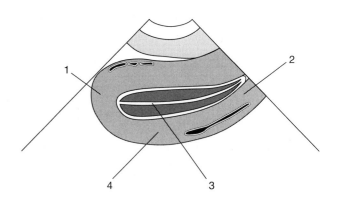

Figure 4–18. Endovaginal sagittal section.

1 _____   3 _____

2 _____   4 _____

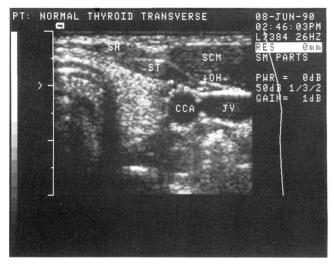

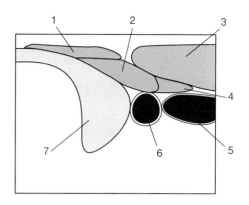

Figure 4–19. Thyroid transverse section.

1 _____   5 _____

2 _____   6 _____

3 _____   7 _____

4 _____

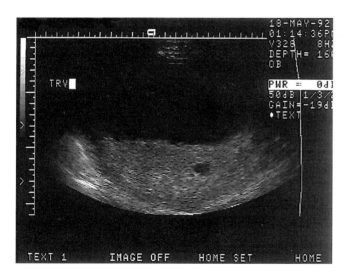

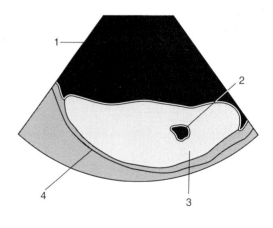

Figure 4–20. Gravid uterus section.

1 _____   3 _____

2 _____   4 _____

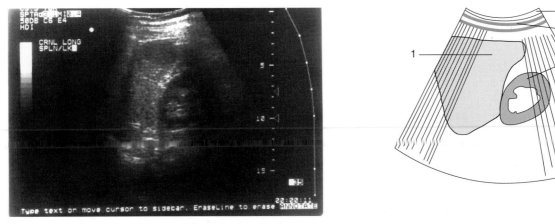

Figure 4–21. Left upper quadrant coronal section.

1 _____   3 _____

2 _____   4 _____

A

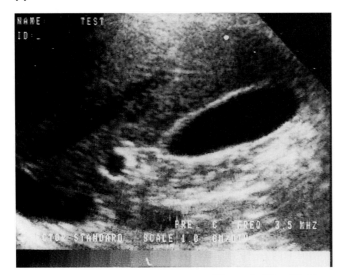
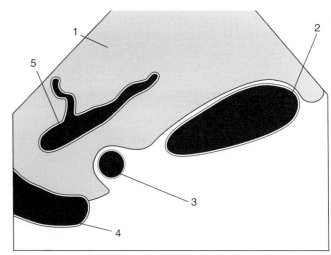

Figure 4–22. Right upper quadrant sagittal section.

1 _____   4 _____

2 _____   5 _____

3 _____

B

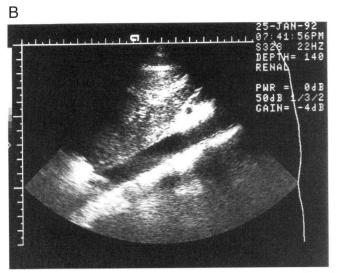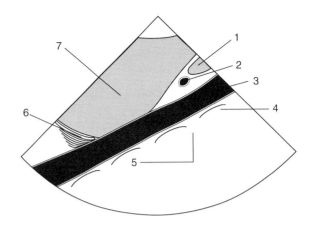

Epigastric sagittal section.

1 _____   5 _____

2 _____   6 _____

3 _____   7 _____

4 _____

C

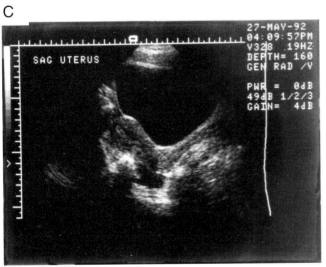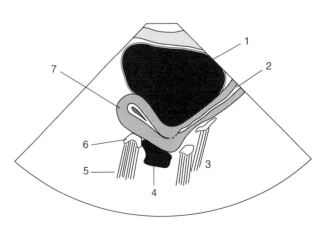

Female pelvis sagittal section.

1 _____   5 _____

2 _____   6 _____

3 _____   7 _____

4 _____

Figure 4–22. *Continued*

D

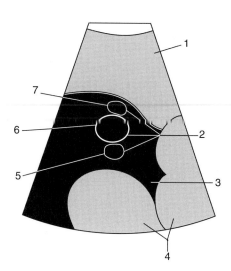

Gravid uterus section.

1 _____   5 _____

2 _____   6 _____

3 _____   7 _____

4 _____

E

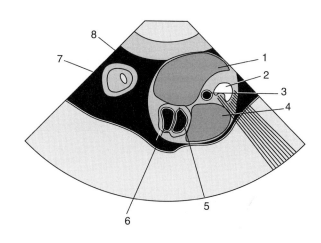

Gravid uterus/fetal abdomen section.

1 _____   5 _____

2 _____   6 _____

3 _____   7 _____

4 _____   8 _____

Figure 4–22. *Continued*

F

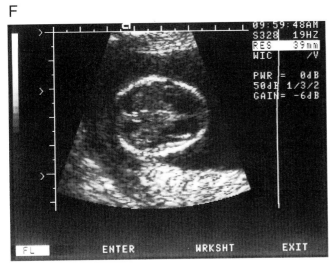
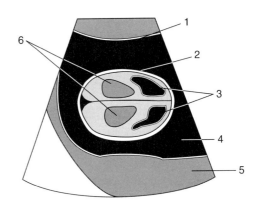

Gravid uterus/fetal head section.

1 _____   4 _____

2 _____   5 _____

3 _____   6 _____

Figure 4–22. *Continued*

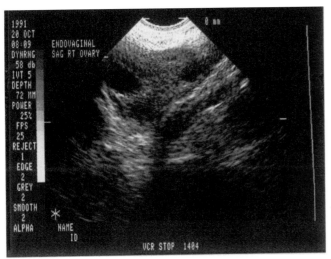
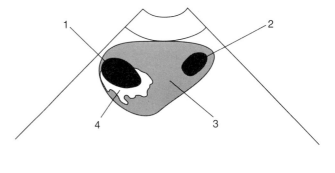

Figure 4–23. Female adnexal endovaginal sagittal section.

1 _____   3 _____

2 _____   4 _____

A

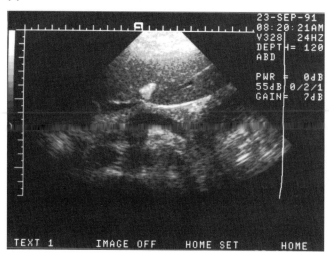
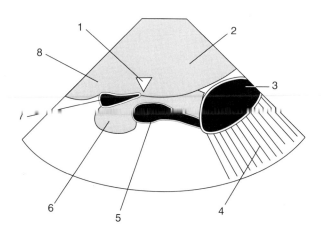

Epigastric transverse section.

1 _____   5 _____

2 _____   6 _____

3 _____   7 _____

4 _____   8 _____

B

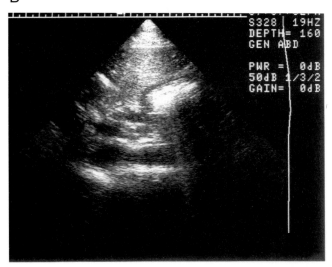
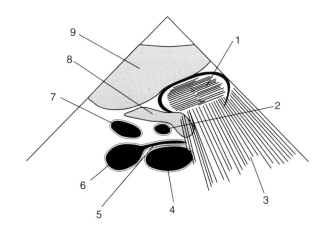

Epigastric transverse section.

1 _____   6 _____

2 _____   7 _____

3 _____   8 _____

4 _____   9 _____

5 _____

Figure 4-24.

A

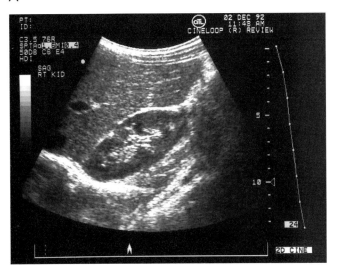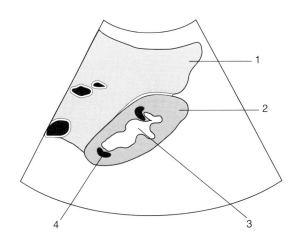

Right upper quadrant sagittal section.

1 _____ 3 _____

2 _____ 4 _____

B

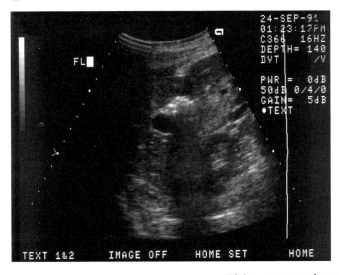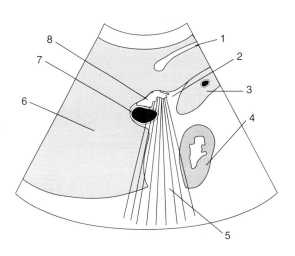

Right upper quadrant transverse section.

1 _____ 5 _____

2 _____ 6 _____

3 _____ 7 _____

4 _____ 8 _____

Figure 4–25.

C

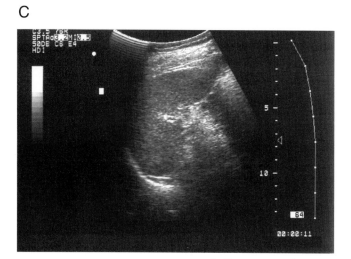 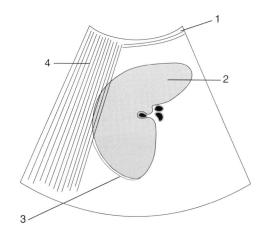

Left upper quadrant coronal section.

1 _____   3 _____

2 _____   4 _____

Figure 4–25. *Continued*

A

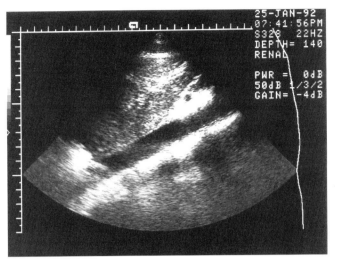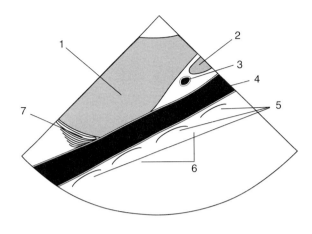

Epigastric sagittal section.

1 _____   5 _____

2 _____   6 _____

3 _____   7 _____

4 _____

B

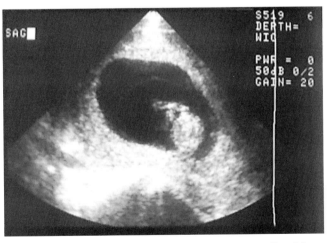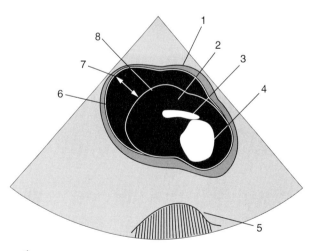

Gravid uterus section.

1 _____   5 _____

2 _____   6 _____

3 _____   7 _____

4 _____   8 _____

Figure 4-26.

C

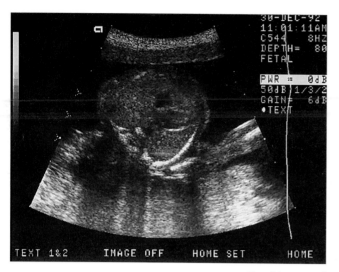 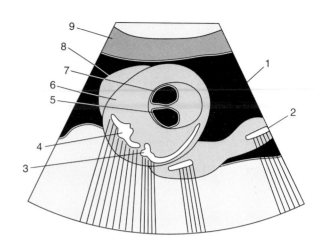

Gravid uterus/fetal thorax section.

1 _____   6 _____

2 _____   7 _____

3 _____   8 _____

4 _____   9 _____

5 _____

D

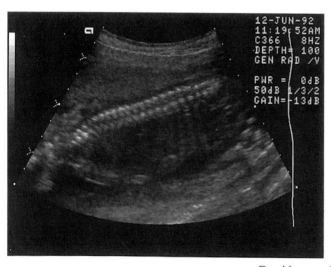 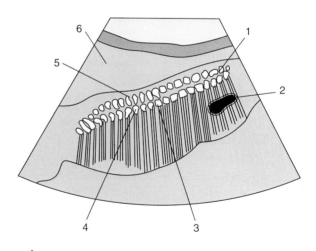

Gravid uterus/fetus section.

1 _____   4 _____

2 _____   5 _____

3 _____   6 _____

Figure 4–26. *Continued*

Chapter 5

THE LIVER

REVIEW QUESTIONS

1. The liver originates from which portion of the primitive gut?

a. foregut

b. hindgut

c. midgut

d. mesentery

2. Any of the following are located within a lobule of the liver, except

a. hepatocytes

b. Küpffer cells

c. portal venules

d. blood sinuses

3. Hemopoiesis is responsible for _____ _____ of the liver.

a. hepatocyte formation

b. the large size

c. the rapid development

d. drainage systems

4. Anomalies of the liver include each of those listed, except:

a. situs inversus

b. hemangioma

c. extrahepatic biliary stenosis

d. Reidel's lobe

5. The surface of the liver which rests upon the abdominal organs is the _____ surface.

a. anterior

b. posterior

c. superior

d. inferior

6. The base of the liver pyramid is the _____ _____ surface.

a. right lateral

b. superior

c. left inferior

d. anterior

7. The caudate lobe of the liver is related to each of the following, except the

a. left portal vein

b. posterior abdominal wall

c. splenic vein

d. inferior vena cava

8. The boundaries of the bare area of the liver include the

a. lesser sac, hepatoduodenal ligament, and the right kidney

b. falciform, coronary, and triangular ligaments

c. inferior vena cava, middle hepatic vein, and main portal vein

d. left coronary ligament, transverse colon, and stomach antrum

9. The liver occupies a major portion of the _____ region.

a. hypogastric

b. umbilical

c. epigastric

d. right hypochondriac

10. The inferior surface of the liver is marked by indentations from each of the following, except

a. hepatic flexure of the colon

b. head of the pancreas

c. right adrenal gland

d. first part of the duodenum

11. The medial portion of the left lobe of the liver is also referred to as the

a. Glisson's cap

b. main lobar fissure

c. papillary projection

d. quadrate lobe

12. The left hepatic lobe is _____ _____ size and shape.

a. fixed in

b. increased, when compared to the right by

c. variable in

d. dependent upon the medial lobe for its

13. Which of the following would result in a false statement? The free inferior margin of the left lobe lies adjacent to the

a. body of the pancreas

b. splenic vein

c. hepatic flexure

d. splenic artery

14. The liver metabolizes

a. fats, carbohydrates, and proteins

b. complex sugars, salts, and bile

c. blood proteins and lymph fluids

d. none of the above

15. The liver is composed of _____ true lobes.

a. two

b. three

c. four

d. five

16. The left hepatic vein and the _____ _____ separate the left hepatic lobe from the caudate.

a. quadrate lobe

b. intersegmental fissure

c. bare area

d. fissure for the ligamentum venosum

17. The hepatic veins are _____ and _____.

a. interlobar

b. intralobar

c. intrasegmental

d. intersegmental

18. The portal system supplies what percentage of total blood flow to the liver?

a. 30

b. 50

c. 75

d. 90

19. The portal confluence has three main tributaries: the inferior mesenteric vein, the superior mesenteric vein, and the

a. middle hepatic vein

b. pancreaticoduodenal vein

c. superior phrenic vein

d. splenic vein

20. The left portal vein communicates with the _____ in patients with severe portal hypertension.

a. right portal vein

b. umbilical vein

c. splenic artery

d. left hepatic vein

21. The caudate lobe is supplied with blood from the

a. right portal vein

b. left portal vein

c. right and left portal veins

d. gastroduodenal artery

22. The opening of the liver through which the portal veins and hepatic arteries enter and through which the hepatic ducts exit is called the

a. portal duct

b. foramen of Winslow

c. porta hepatis

d. greater omentum

23. The common bile duct and the hepatic artery course _____ to the portal vein within the liver.

   a. anterior

   b. medial

   c. superior

   d. posterior

24. The liver should have a(an) _____ _____ sonographic appearance.

   a. anechoic

   b. homogeneous

   c. heterogeneous

   d. low level echogenicity in its

25. The main lobar fissure represents a

   a. landmark for the caudate lobe

   b. divider between the mid and lateral portions of the left lobe

   c. marker for the falciform ligament

   d. boundary between the right and left lobes

26. The left portal vein takes a c-shaped superior course in the liver, proximal to the

   a. falciform ligament

   b. caudate lobe

   c. left hepatic vein

   d. ligamentum venosum

27. A fibrous cord which extends upward from the diaphragm to the anterior wall and was patent before birth may be noted as any of the following except the

   a. round ligament

   b. ligamentum teres

   c. falciform ligament

   d. umbilical vein

28. The hepatic veins _____ in size as they drain toward the IVC.

   a. increase

   b. decrease

   c. do not change

29. Abnormal lesions usually are _____ _____ in echogenicity when compared to the moderate echo strength of the liver parenchyma.

   a. increased

   b. decreased

   c. either increased or decreased

   d. similar

30. Normal variants of the liver include a right lobe which may extend inferiorly to the iliac crest or a left lobe which may extend laterally to the spleen.

   a. true

   b. false

   c. do not change

Identify the structures indicated in the following illustrations. These figures duplicate those found in **ULTRASONOGRAPHY: Introduction to Normal Structure and Functional Anatomy**. Refer to the textbook if you need help.

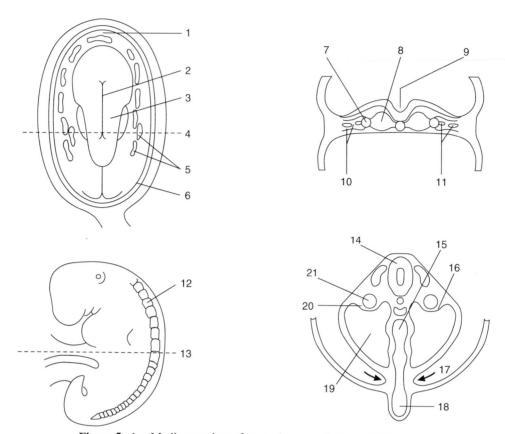

Figure 5-1. Median section of an embryo outlining primitive gut.

1 _____   12 _____

2 _____   13 _____

3 _____   14 _____

4 _____   15 _____

5 _____   16 _____

6 _____   17 _____

7 _____   18 _____

8 _____   19 _____

9 _____   20 _____

10 _____   21 _____

11 _____

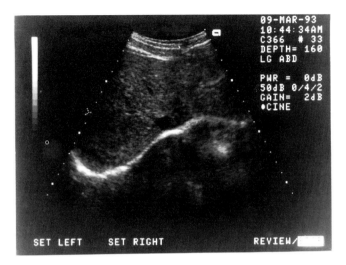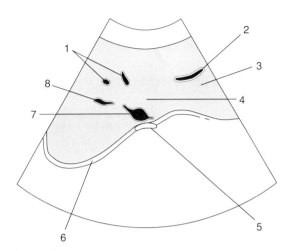

Figure 5-2. Posterosuperior liver surface.

1 _____   5 _____

2 _____   6 _____

3 _____   7 _____

4 _____   8 _____

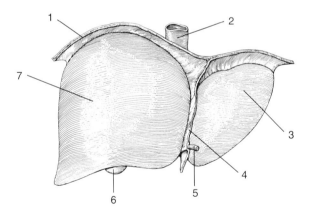

Figure 5-3. Anterior liver surface.

1 _____

2 _____

3 _____

4 _____

5 _____

6 _____

7 _____

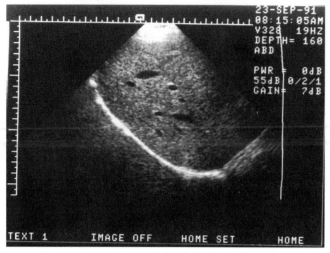 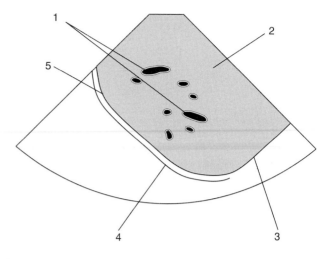

Figure 5-4. Longitudinal scan of right lateral margin of liver.

1 _____   4 _____

2 _____   5 _____

3 _____

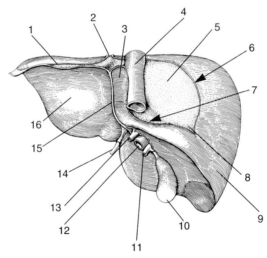

Figure 5-5. Posterior liver surface.

1 _____   9 _____

2 _____   10 _____

3 _____   11 _____

4 _____   12 _____

5 _____   13 _____

6 _____   14 _____

7 _____   15 _____

8 _____   16 _____

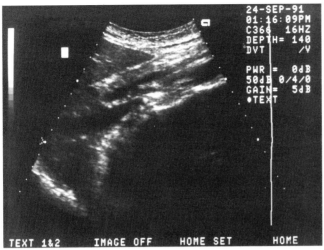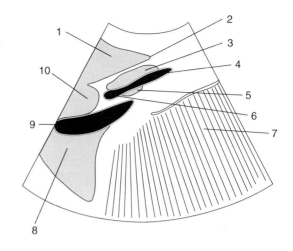

Figure 5–6. Longitudinal image of left inferior margin of left hepatic lobe.

1 _____   6 _____
2 _____   7 _____
3 _____   8 _____
4 _____   9 _____
5 _____   10 _____

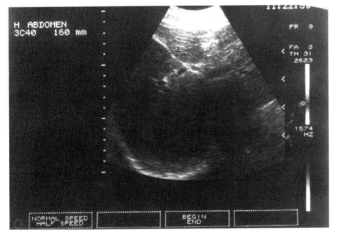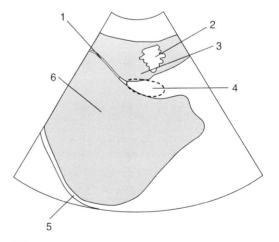

Figure 5–7. Transverse scan of liver.

1 _____   4 _____
2 _____   5 _____
3 _____   6 _____

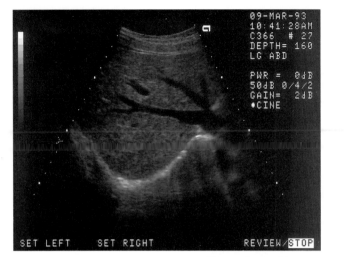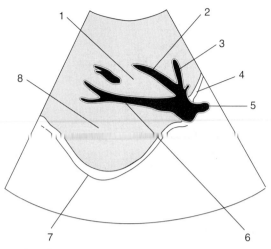

Figure 5-8. Transverse scan of hepatic veins.

1 _____   5 _____

2 _____   6 _____

3 _____   7 _____

4 _____   8 _____

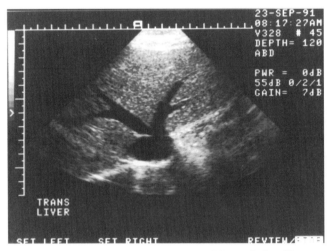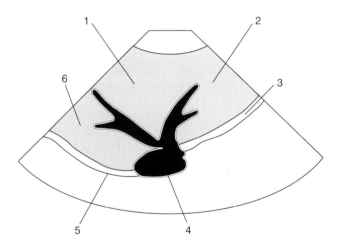

Figure 5-9. Transverse scan of hepatic veins.

1 _____   4 _____

2 _____   5 _____

3 _____   6 _____

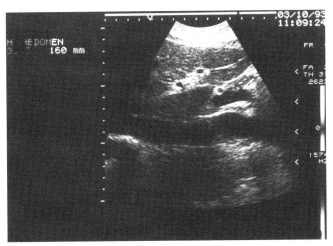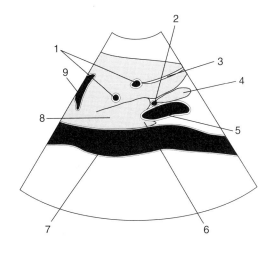

Figure 5-10. Longitudinal image of main portal vein.

1 _____   6 _____

2 _____   7 _____

3 _____   8 _____

4 _____   9 _____

5 _____

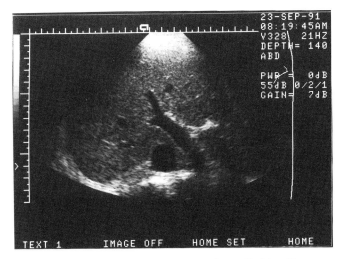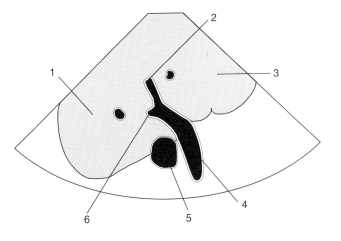

Figure 5-11. Transverse image of main portal vein.

1 _____   4 _____

2 _____   5 _____

3 _____   6 _____

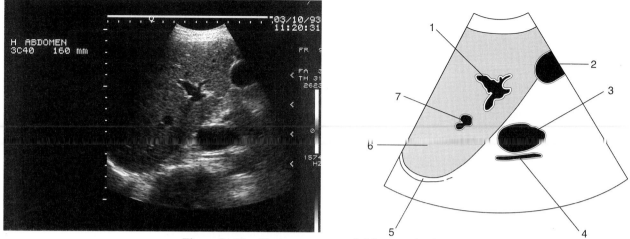

Figure 5–12. Transverse scan of right portal vein.

1 _____   5 _____

2 _____   6 _____

3 _____   7 _____

4 _____

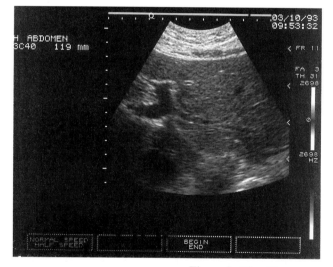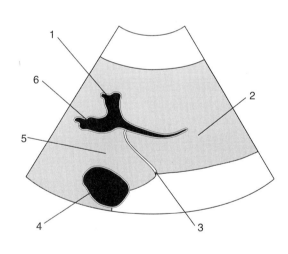

Figure 5–13. Transverse scan of portal vein branches.

1 _____   4 _____

2 _____   5 _____

3 _____   6 _____

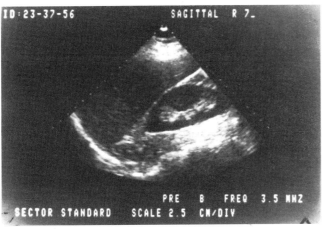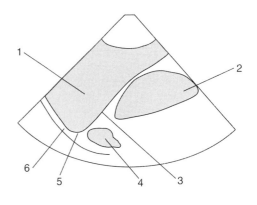

Figure 5–14. Longitudinal scan of bare area of the liver.

1 _____   4 _____

2 _____   5 _____

3 _____   6 _____

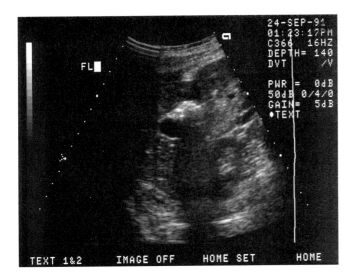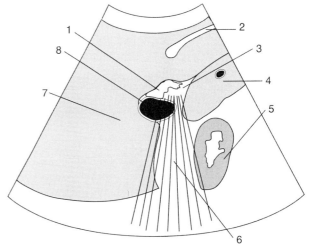

Figure 5–15. Longitudinal scan of falciform ligament.

1 _____   5 _____

2 _____   6 _____

3 _____   7 _____

4 _____   8 _____

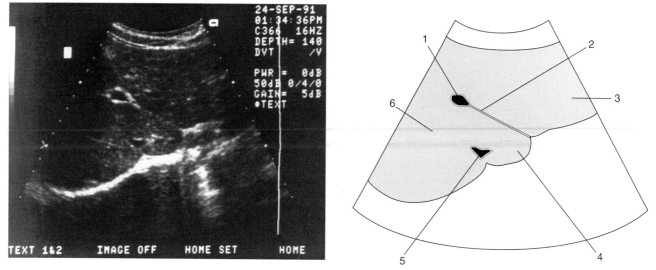

Figure 5–16. Transverse scan of the caudate lobe.

1 _____   4 _____

2 _____   5 _____

3 _____   6 _____

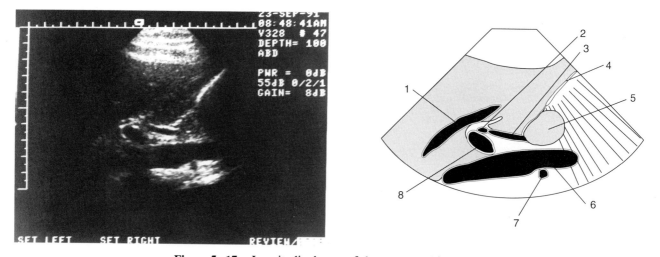

Figure 5–17. Longitudinal scan of the common bile duct.

1 _____   5 _____

2 _____   6 _____

3 _____   7 _____

4 _____   8 _____

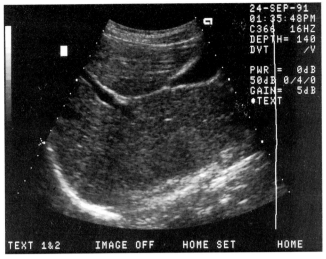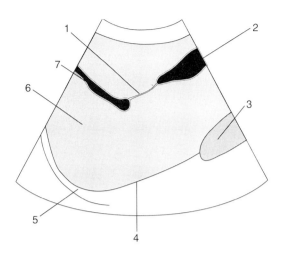

Figure 5–18. Longitudinal scan of the main lobar fissure.

1 _____   5 _____

2 _____   6 _____

3 _____   7 _____

4 _____

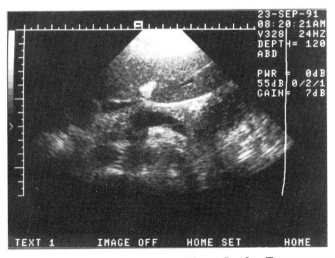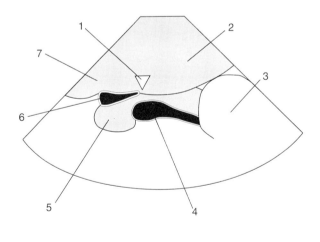

Figure 5–19. Transverse scan of the falciform ligament.

1 _____   5 _____

2 _____   6 _____

3 _____   7 _____

4 _____

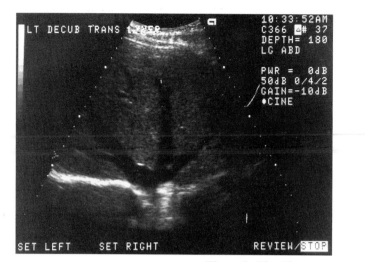
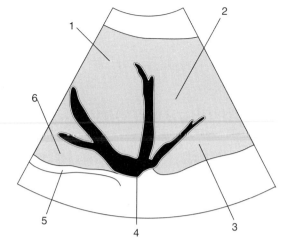

Figure 5-20. Transverse scan of hepatic lobes.

1 _____   4 _____

2 _____   5 _____

3 _____   6 _____

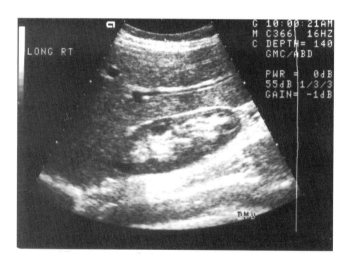
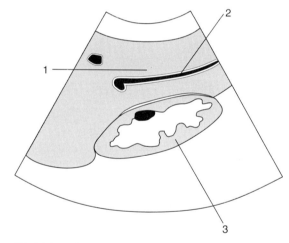

Figure 5-23. Longitudinal image of Reidel's lobe.

1 _____

2 _____

3 _____

Chapter 6

THE BILIARY SYSTEM

REVIEW QUESTIONS

1. The gallbladder is located _____ _____ and _____ to the liver.

  a. anterior and medial

  b. anterior and right lateral

  c. posterior and inferior

  d. posterior and superior

2. The porta hepatis is

  a. a normal variant of the liver

  b. the hilum or doorway to the liver

  c. the area of the liver that the inferior vena cava passes through

  d. the name of the liver fossa in the right upper quadrant

3. The proximal portion of the biliary duct is the

  a. common hepatic duct

  b. cystic duct

  c. common bile duct

  d. supraduodenal portion of the common bile duct

4. The intrahepatic ducts are the

  a. common hepatic duct and cystic duct

  b. common hepatic duct and common bile duct

  c. cystic duct and common bile duct

  d. right and left hepatic ducts

5. The distal portion of the biliary duct is the

  a. common bile duct

  b. common hepatic duct

  c. cystic duct

  d. main portal vein.

6. The portal triad consists of the

  a. portal vein, hepatic vein, and common bile duct

  b. portal vein, hepatic artery, and common bile duct

  c. portal vein, hepatic artery, and common bile duct

  d. portal vein, hepatic vein, and common hepatic duct

7. The range of normal diameter size of the common hepatic and common bile ducts is

  a. 1 mm to 5 mm

  b. 5 mm to 10 mm

  c. 1 mm to 7 mm

  d. 4 mm to 6 mm

8. The normal thickness of the gallbladder wall is

  a. .5 mm

  b. 3 mm or less

  c. 6 mm

  d. 1 mm or less

9. In most cases the fundus of the gallbladder is located _____ to the superior pole of the right kidney.

  a. right lateral

  b. posterior

  c. medial

  d. anterior

10. The bile-filled biliary system can be described sonographically as

  a. hyperechoic

  b. anechoic with echogenic walls

  c. hypoechoic

  d. having medium to low level echoes with reflective walls

Identify the structures indicated in the following illustrations. These figures duplicate those found in **ULTRASONOGRAPHY: Introduction to Normal Structure and Functional Anatomy**. Refer to the textbook if you need help.

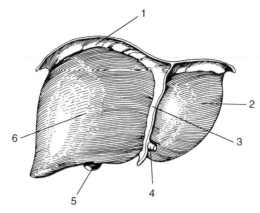

Figure 6-1. Location of gallbladder in relationship to anterior view of liver.

1 _____   4 _____

2 _____   5 _____

3 _____   6 _____

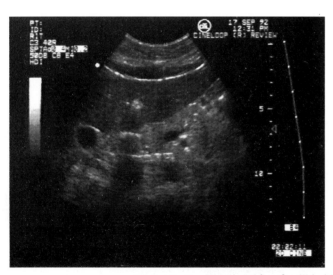 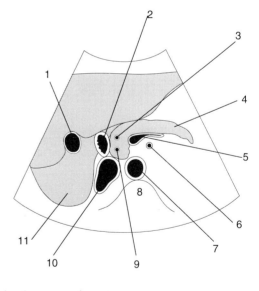

Figure 6-2. Relationship of gallbladder, duodenum, and pancreas.

1 _____   7 _____

2 _____   8 _____

3 _____   9 _____

4 _____   10 _____

5 _____   11 _____

6 _____

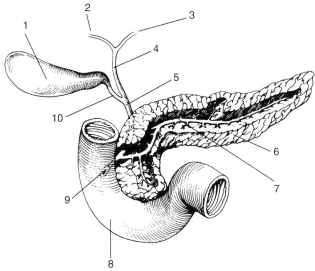

Figure 6–3. Biliary system, including pancreas and pancreatic duct.

1 _____   6 _____

2 _____   7 _____

3 _____   8 _____

4 _____   9 _____

5 _____   10 _____

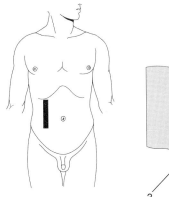
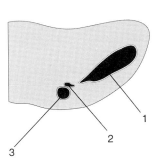
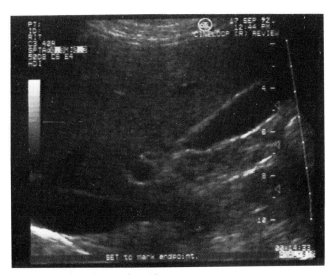

Figure 6–4. Common hepatic duct and portal vein relationship.

1 _____

2 _____

3 _____

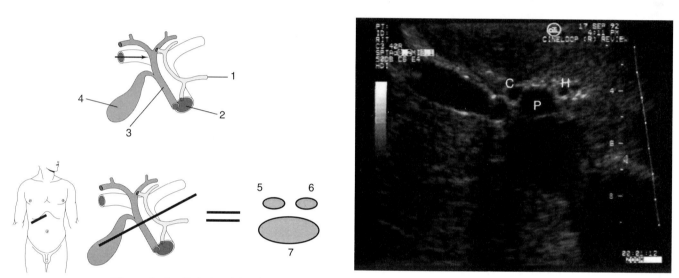

Figure 6–5. Relationship of the portal vein to the hepatic artery and common bile duct.

1 _____   5 _____

2 _____   6 _____

3 _____   7 _____

4 _____

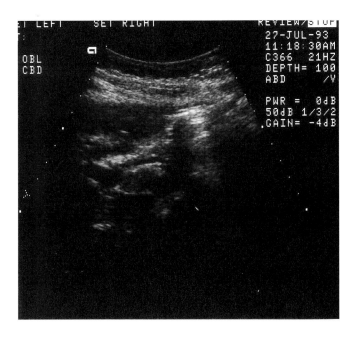
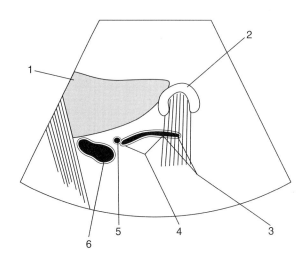

1 _____   4 _____

2 _____   5 _____

3 _____   6 _____

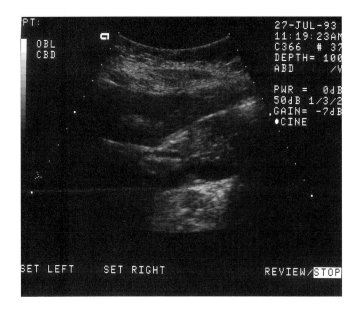
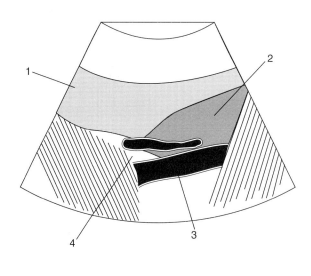

1 _____   3 _____

2 _____   4 _____

Figure 6-6. *Top* and *bottom*, Longitudinal sections of the common bile duct.

Ultrasound images courtesy of Jeanes Hospital, Philadelphia, PA.

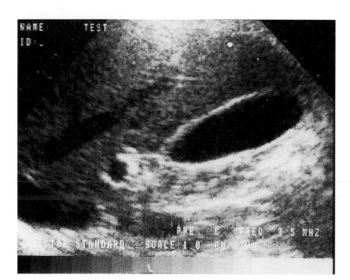 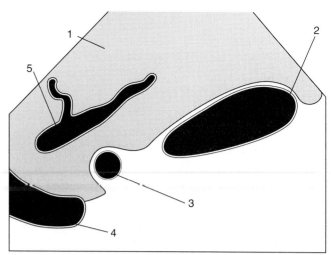

Figure 6-7. Longitudinal section of gallbladder.

1 _____   4 _____

2 _____   5 _____

3 _____

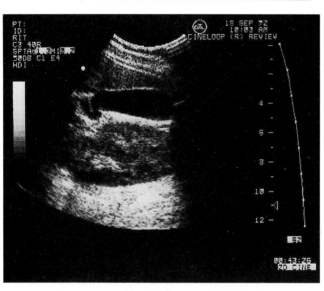 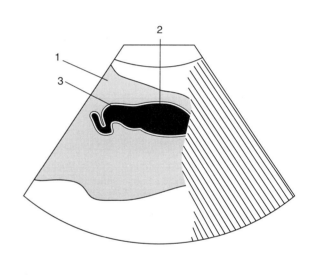

Figure 6-8. Longitudinal section of gallbladder.

1 _____

2 _____

3 _____

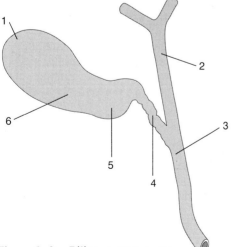

Figure 6-9. Biliary system anatomy.

82

1 _____

2 _____

3 _____

4 _____

5 _____

6 _____

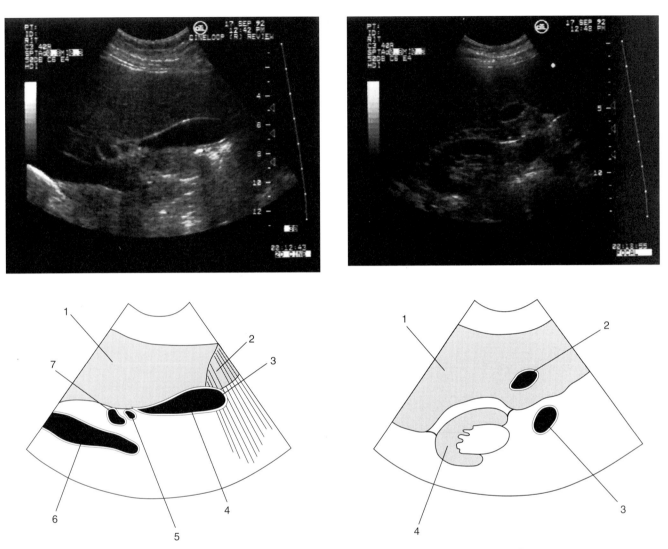

Figure 6-10. *Left,* Longitudinal section of gallbladder; *right,* Transverse section of gallbladder.

1 _____   1 _____

2 _____   2 _____

3 _____   3 _____

4 _____   4 _____

5 _____

6 _____

7 _____

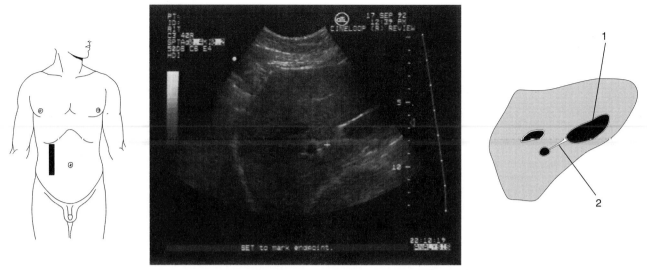

Figure 6–12. Relationship of gallbladder to main lobar fissure.

1 _____

2 _____

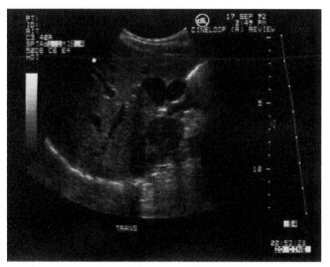

Figure 6–14. Longitudinal section of gallbladder.

1 _____ 3 _____

2 _____ 4 _____

1 _____

2 _____

3 _____

4 _____

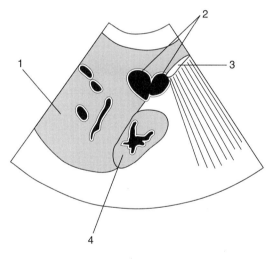

Figure 6–15. Gallbladder variations.

THE PANCREAS

REVIEW QUESTIONS

1. Name the parts of the pancreas and the vascular anatomy which borders it.

2. Name the blood supply to the pancreas.

3. List three components of pancreatic juice and the food substances they act upon.

4. List three hormones produced by the pancreas and their function.

5. List two structures which appear in the head of the pancreas. How can you identify these structures on images?

6. Describe the echogenicity of the pancreas.

7. On a transverse image of the pancreas, what type of section of the pancreas can be obtained?

8. A sagittal image shows the aorta and superior mesenteric artery. What part of the pancreas will be shown?

9. What part of the pancreas is located to the left (toward the aorta) of an imaginary line drawn between the portal/splenic confluence and the inferior vena cava?

10. Describe vessels from the biliary tree and pancreas which enter the duodenum.

Identify the structures indicated in the illustrations which are shown on the following pages. These figures duplicate those found in **ULTRASONOGRAPHY: Introduction to Normal Structure and Functional Anatomy**. Refer to the textbook if you need help.

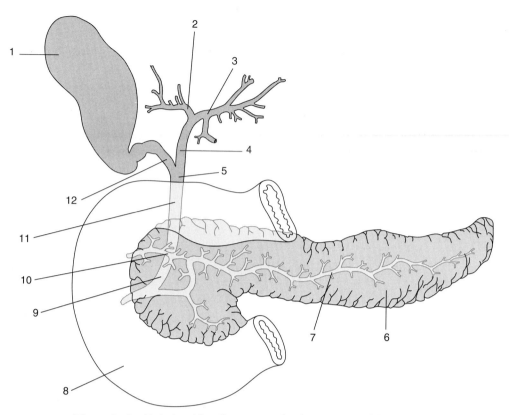

Figure 7–1. Relationship of pancreas, duodenum, and biliary system.

1 _____   7 _____

2 _____   8 _____

3 _____   9 _____

4 _____   10 _____

5 _____   11 _____

6 _____   12 _____

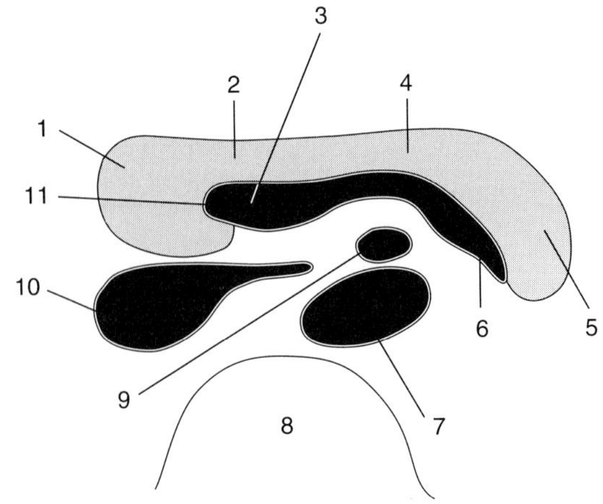

1 _____

2 _____

3 _____

4 _____

5 _____

6 _____

7 _____

8 _____

9 _____

Figure 7–2. The portal/splenic confluence.

10 _____

11 _____

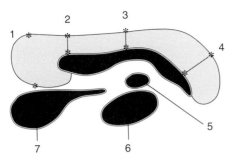

Figure 7–3. Caliper placement for measuring the pancreas.

1 _____

2 _____

3 _____

4 _____

5 _____

6 _____

7 _____

1 _____

2 _____

3 _____

4 _____

5 _____

6 _____

7 _____

8 _____

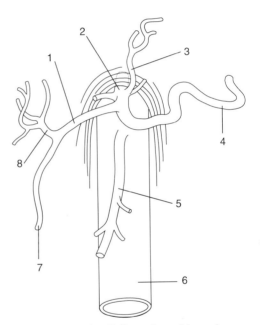

Figure 7–4. Celiac axis and branches.

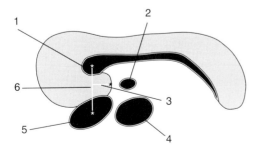

Figure 7–5. Transverse view of uncinate process.

1 _____

2 _____

3 _____

4 _____

5 _____

6 _____

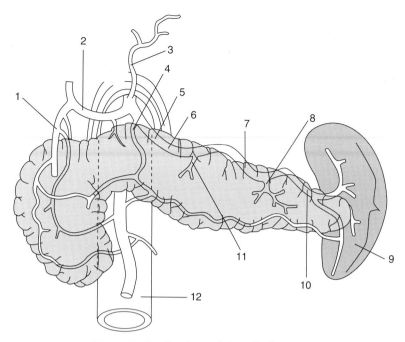

Figure 7–6. Sections of the splenic artery.

1 _____

2 _____

3 _____

4 _____

5 _____

6 _____

7 _____

8 _____

9 _____

10 _____

11 _____

12 _____

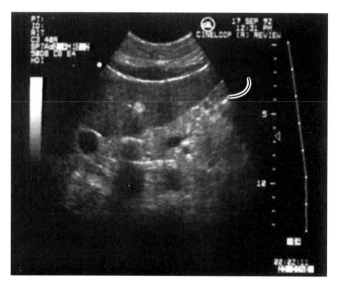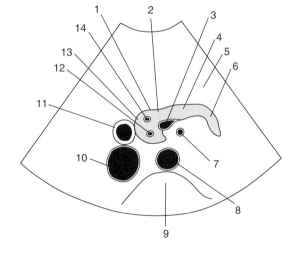

Figure 7–7. Transverse image of the pancreas.

1 _____   8 _____

2 _____   9 _____

3 _____   10 _____

4 _____   11 _____

5 _____   12 _____

6 _____   13 _____

7 _____   14 _____

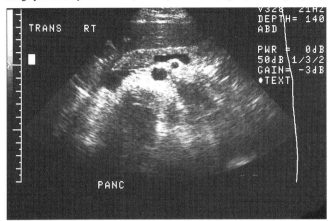 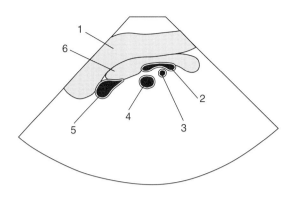

Figure 7-8. Transverse image of the pancreas.

1 _____ 4 _____

2 _____ 5 _____

3 _____ 6 _____

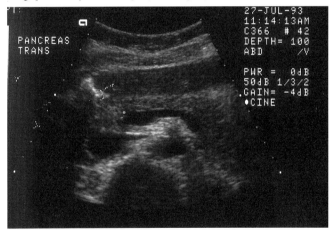 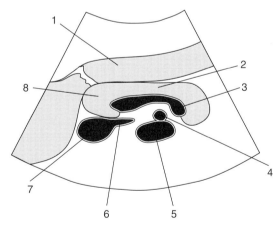

Figure 7-9. Transverse image of the pancreas.

1 _____ 5 _____

2 _____ 6 _____

3 _____ 7 _____

4 _____ 8 _____

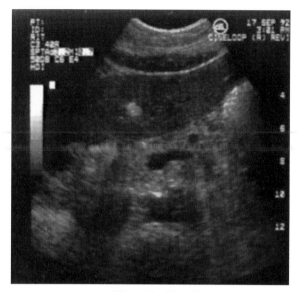 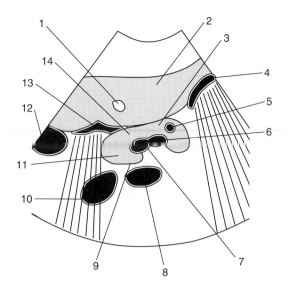

Figure 7–10. Transverse image showing a longitudinal section of the pancreas.

1 _____	8 _____	
2 _____	9 _____	
3 _____	10 _____	
4 _____	11 _____	
5 _____	12 _____	
6 _____	13 _____	
7 _____	14 _____	

Image provided by Jeanes Hospital, Philadelphia, PA.

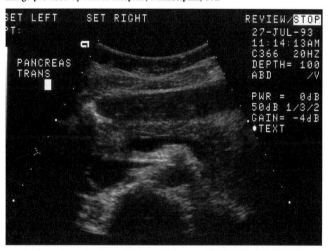 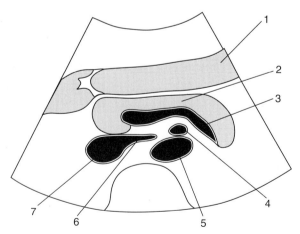

Figure 7–11. Transverse image of the pancreas.

1 _____	5 _____
2 _____	6 _____
3 _____	7 _____
4 _____	

Image provided by Jeanes Hospital, Philadelphia, PA.

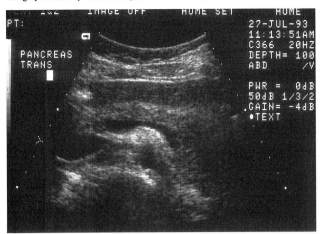 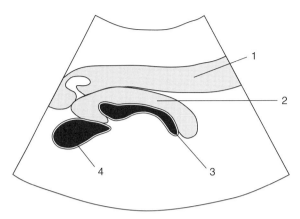

Figure 7–12. Transverse image of the pancreas.

1 _____   3 _____

2 _____   4 _____

Image provided by Rose Merna-Weston, RDMS, Nazareth Hospital, Philadelphia, PA.

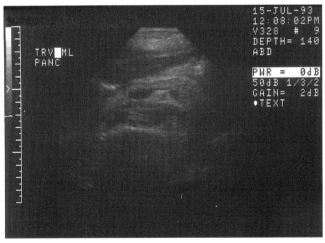 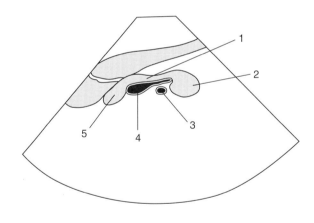

Figure 7–13. Transverse image of the pancreas.

1 _____   4 _____

2 _____   5 _____

3 _____

Image provided by Jeanes Hospital, Philadelphia, PA.

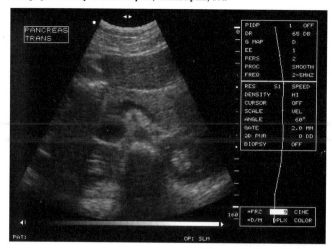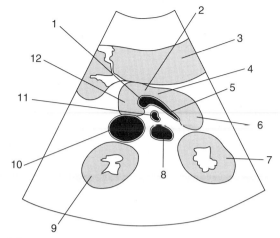

Figure 7–14. Transverse image of the pancreas.

1 _____   7 _____

2 _____   8 _____

3 _____   9 _____

4 _____   10 _____

5 _____   11 _____

6 _____   12 _____

Image provided by Carol Prives, RDMS, Nazareth Hospital, Philadelphia, PA.

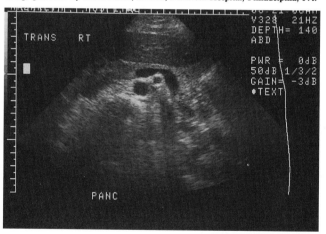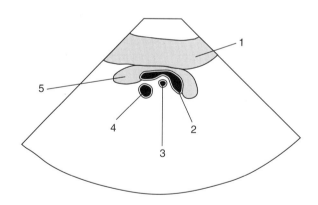

Figure 7–15. Transverse image of the pancreas.

1 _____   4 _____

2 _____   5 _____

3 _____

Image provided by Jeanes Hospital, Philadelphia, PA.

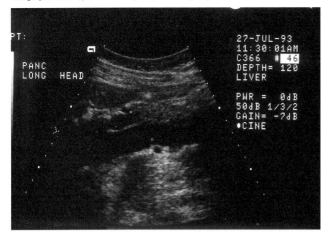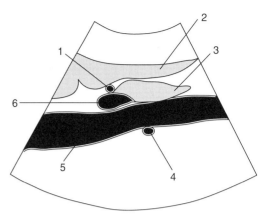

Figure 7–16. Sagittal image of pancreas head.

1 _____   4 _____

2 _____   5 _____

3 _____   6 _____

Image provided by Jeanes Hospital, Philadelphia, PA.

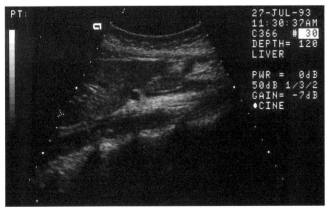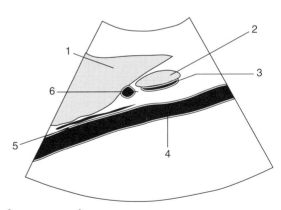

Figure 7–17. Sagittal image of pancreas neck.

1 _____   4 _____

2 _____   5 _____

3 _____   6 _____

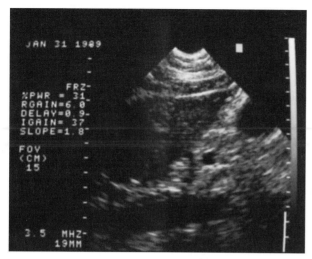 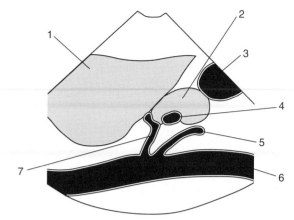

Figure 7–18. Sagittal image of pancreas body.

1 _____   5 _____

2 _____   6 _____

3 _____   7 _____

4 _____

Image provided by Jeanes Hospital, Philadelphia, PA.

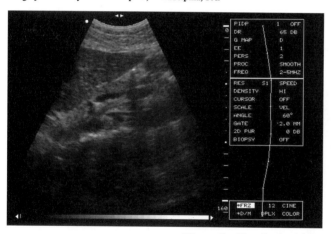 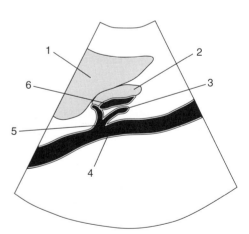

Figure 7–19. Sagittal image of pancreas body.

1 _____   4 _____

2 _____   5 _____

3 _____   6 _____

Image provided by Jeanes Hospital, Philadelphia, PA.

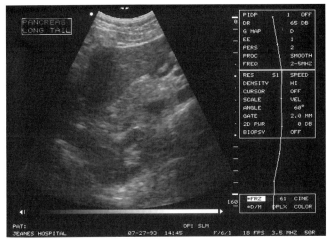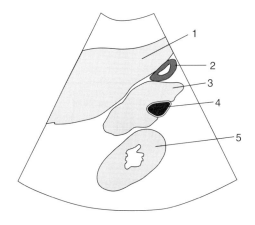

Figure 7-20. Sagittal image of pancreas tail.

1 _____   4 _____

2 _____   5 _____

3 _____

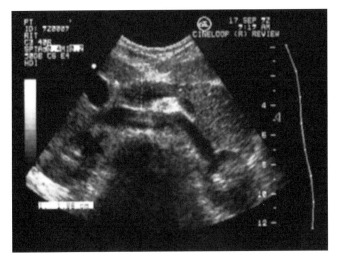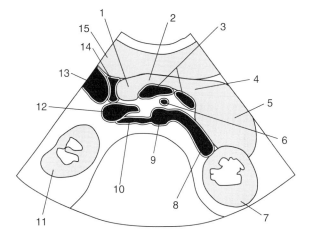

Figure 7-21. Transverse image of the pancreas.

1 _____   9 _____

2 _____   10 _____

3 _____   11 _____

4 _____   12 _____

5 _____   13 _____

6 _____   14 _____

7 _____   15 _____

8 _____

Chapter 8

THE URINARY SYSTEM

REVIEW QUESTIONS

1. Describe the function of the urinary system.

2. The kidneys are anterior to which structures?

3. The right kidney is posterior to which structures?

4. The left kidney is posterior to which structures?

5. Describe the location of the ureters.

6. Describe the location of the urinary bladder.

7. List the normal sizes of the urinary system structures.

8. Describe urine development by the kidneys.

9. Describe the parts of the urinary system and their sonographic appearance.

10. List the reasons why ultrasound is used to evaluate the urinary system.

11. Describe the normal variants of the urinary system that are recognized by ultrasound.

12. Name three types of physicians who diagnose or treat the urinary system and define what they do.

13. Name and define two diagnostic tests other than ultrasound that are commonly used to evaluate the urinary system.

14. What are the normal laboratory values for BUN and Cr, and what do these values represent?

15. Name and define the hormones that affect the kidneys.

Identify the structures indicated in the illustrations which are shown on the following pages. These figures duplicate those found in **ULTRASONOGRAPHY: Introduction to Normal Structure and Functional Anatomy**. Refer to the textbook if you need help.

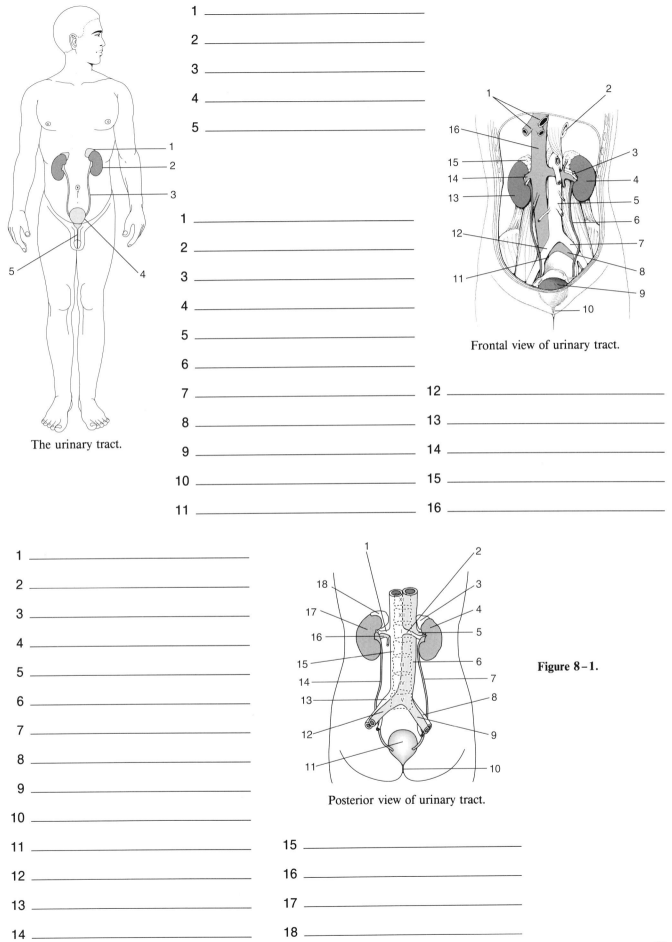

The urinary tract.

Frontal view of urinary tract.

Posterior view of urinary tract.

Figure 8–1.

1 _____
2 _____
3 _____
4 _____
5 _____

1 _____
2 _____
3 _____
4 _____
5 _____
6 _____
7 _____
8 _____
9 _____
10 _____
11 _____

12 _____
13 _____
14 _____
15 _____
16 _____

1 _____
2 _____
3 _____
4 _____
5 _____
6 _____
7 _____
8 _____
9 _____
10 _____
11 _____
12 _____
13 _____
14 _____

15 _____
16 _____
17 _____
18 _____

1 _____

2 _____

3 _____

4 _____

5 _____

6 _____

7 _____

8 _____

9 _____

10 _____

11 _____

12 _____

13 _____

14 _____

15 _____

16 _____

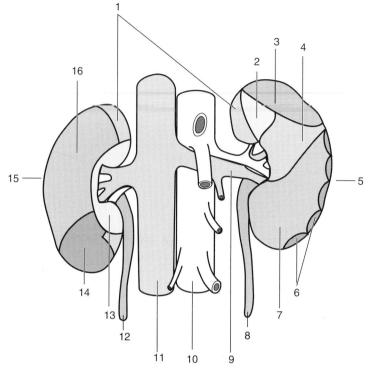

Figure 8–2. Anterior view of kidneys. Shaded areas indicate overlying structures.

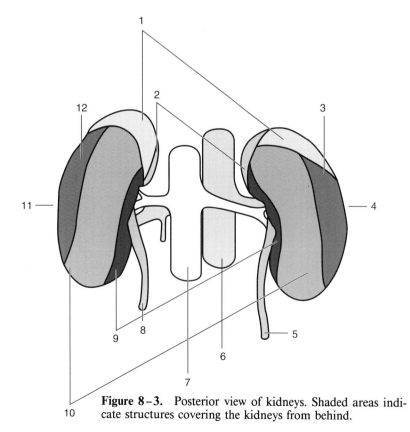

Figure 8–3. Posterior view of kidneys. Shaded areas indicate structures covering the kidneys from behind.

1 _____

2 _____

3 _____

4 _____

5 _____

6 _____

7 _____

8 _____

9 _____

10 _____

11 _____

12 _____

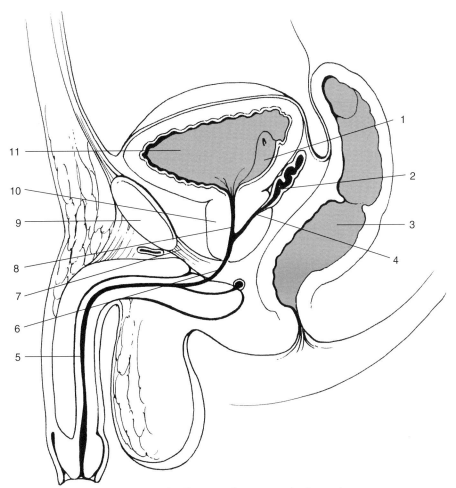

Figure 8–4. Lower urinary tract in the male.

1 _____   7 _____

2 _____   8 _____

3 _____   9 _____

4 _____   10 _____

5 _____   11 _____

6 _____

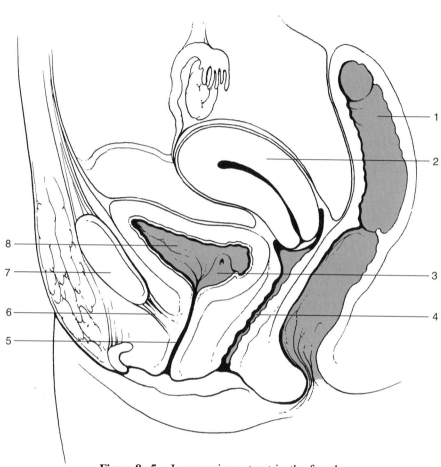

Figure 8-5. Lower urinary tract in the female.

1 _____   5 _____

2 _____   6 _____

3 _____   7 _____

4 _____   8 _____

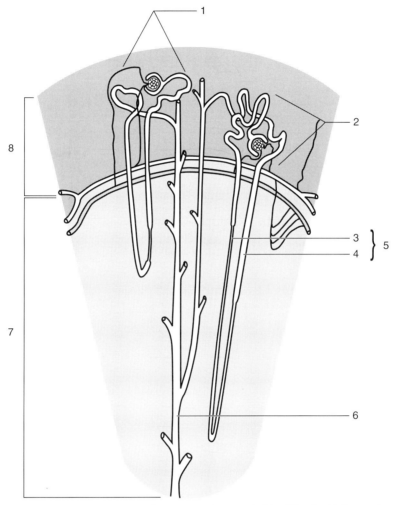

Figure 8–6. Cortical and juxtamedullary nephritis. (Fig. 8–11 in text.)

1 _____   5 _____

2 _____   6 _____

3 _____   7 _____

4 _____   8 _____

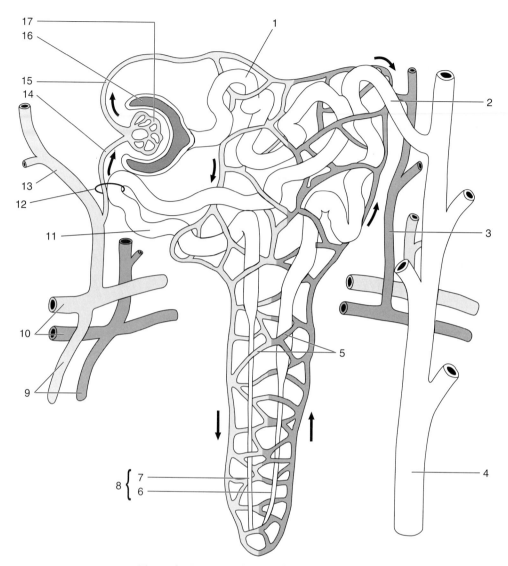

Figure 8–7. A nephron. (Fig. 8–12 in text.)

1 _____	10 _____
2 _____	11 _____
3 _____	12 _____
4 _____	13 _____
5 _____	14 _____
6 _____	15 _____
7 _____	16 _____
8 _____	17 _____
9 _____	

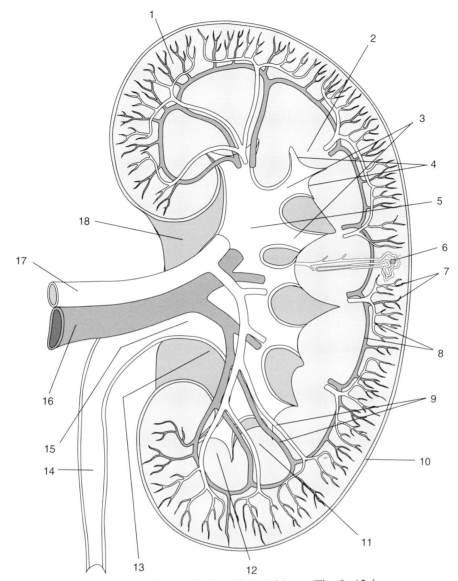

Figure 8–8. Dissected view of the kidney. (Fig. 8–13 in text.)

1 _____

2 _____

3 _____

4 _____

5 _____

6 _____

7 _____

8 _____

9 _____

10 _____

11 _____

12 _____

13 _____

14 _____

15 _____

16 _____

17 _____

18 _____

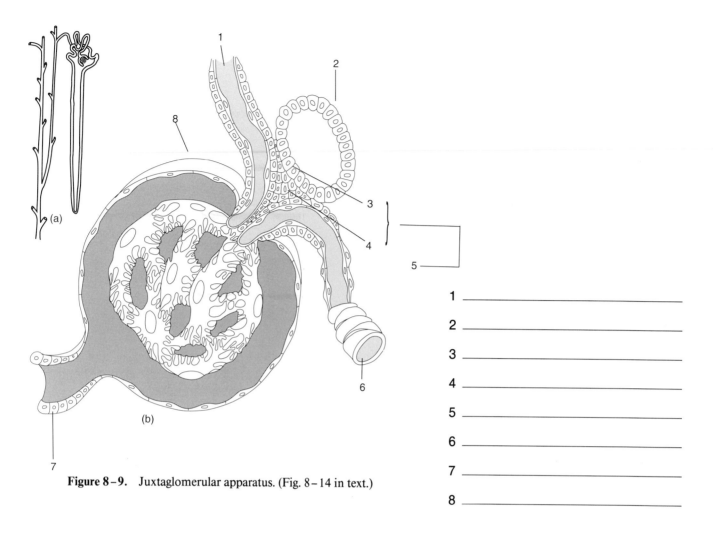

Figure 8-9. Juxtaglomerular apparatus. (Fig. 8-14 in text.)

1 _____
2 _____
3 _____
4 _____
5 _____
6 _____
7 _____
8 _____

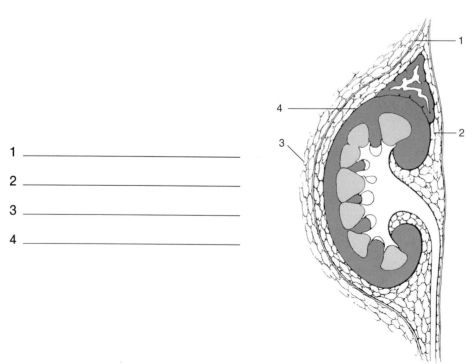

1 _____
2 _____
3 _____
4 _____

Figure 8-10. Four layers surrounding the kidney. (Fig. 8-6 in text.)

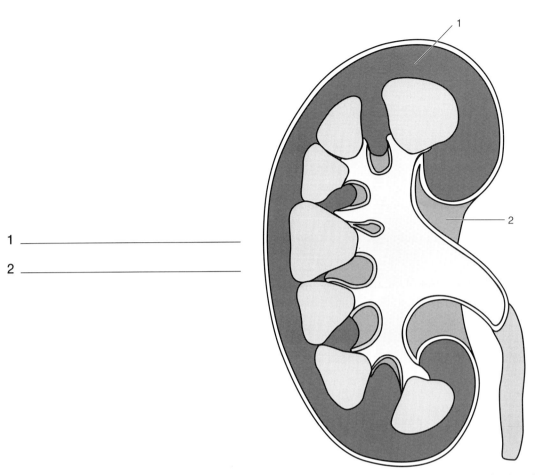

1 _____

2 _____

Figure 8–11. Kidney parenchyma and sinus. (Fig. 8–7 in text.)

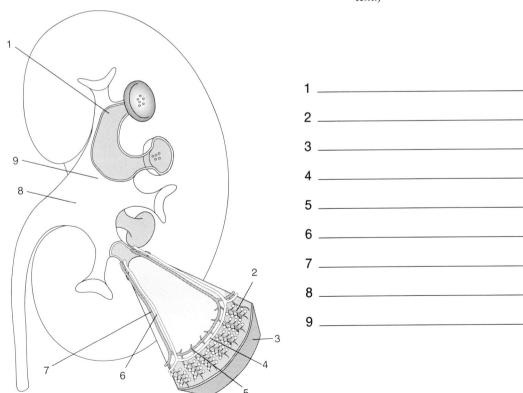

Figure 8–12. Renal lobe. (Fig. 8–8 in text.)

1 _____

2 _____

3 _____

4 _____

5 _____

6 _____

7 _____

8 _____

9 _____

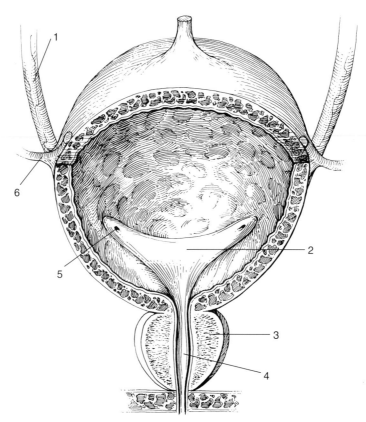

Figure 8–13. Urinary bladder. (Fig. 8–9 in text.)

1 _____   4 _____

2 _____   5 _____

3 _____   6 _____

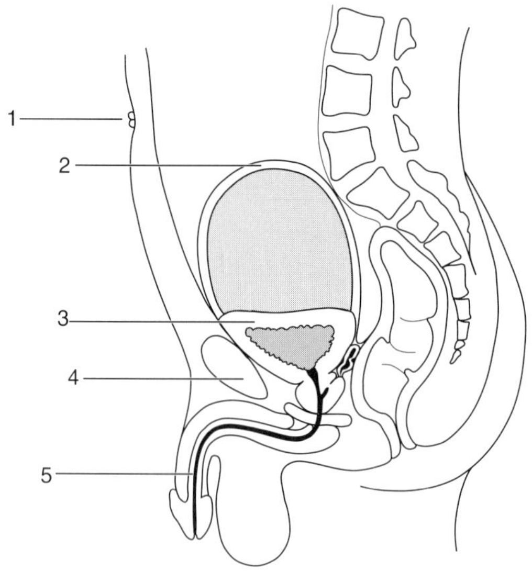

Figure 8–14. Difference between an empty and a distended bladder. (Fig. 8–10 in text.)

1 _____   4 _____

2 _____   5 _____

3 _____

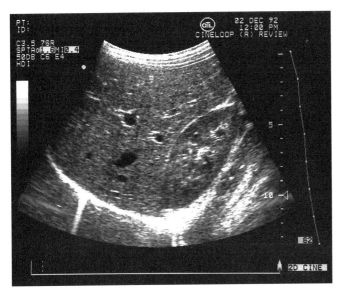
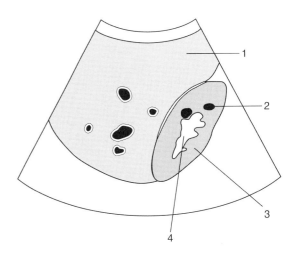

Figure 8–15. Sagittal right kidney.

1 _____   3 _____

2 _____   4 _____

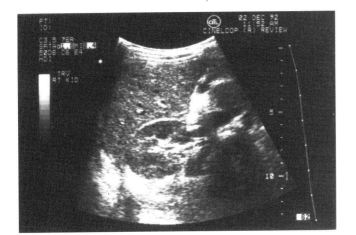
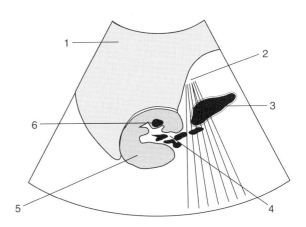

Figure 8–16. Transverse right kidney.

1 _____   4 _____

2 _____   5 _____

3 _____   6 _____

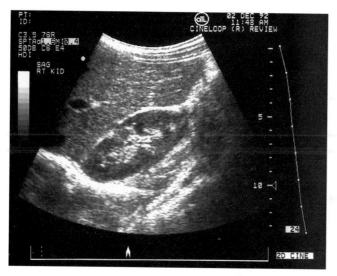
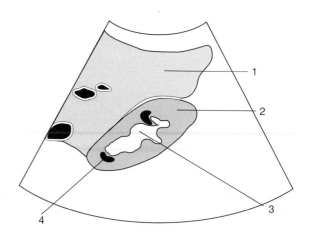

Figure 8–17. Sagittal right kidney.

1 _____   3 _____

2 _____   4 _____

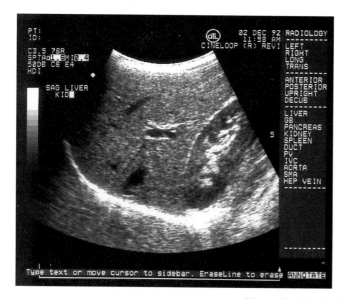
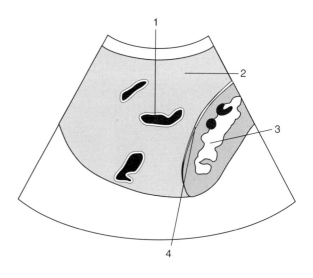

Figure 8–18. Sagittal right kidney.

1 _____   3 _____

2 _____   4 _____

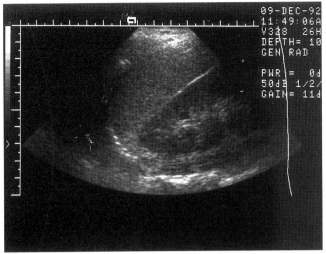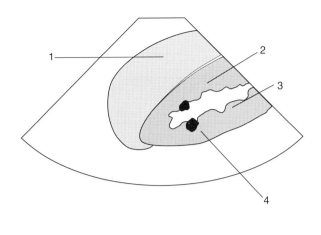

Figure 8–19. Coronal left kidney and spleen.

1 _____   3 _____

2 _____   4 _____

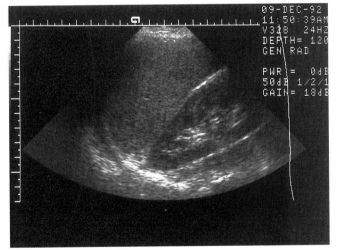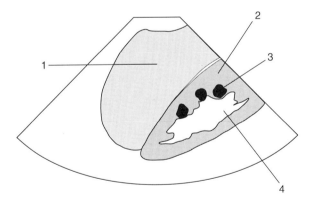

Figure 8–20. Coronal left kidney and spleen.

1 _____   3 _____

2 _____   4 _____

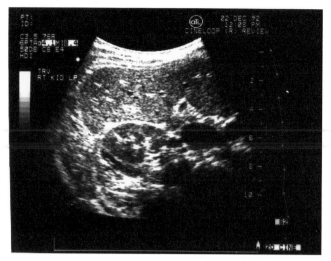
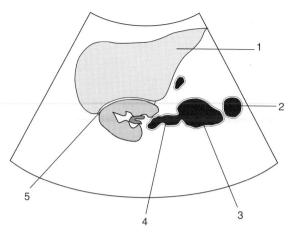

Figure 8–21. Transverse liver and right kidney.

1 _____   4 _____

2 _____   5 _____

3 _____

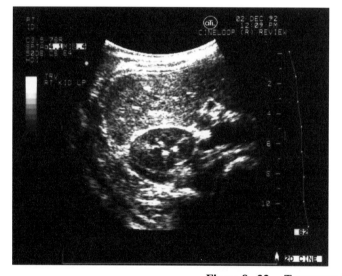
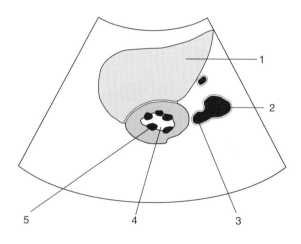

Figure 8–22. Transverse liver and right kidney.

1 _____   4 _____

2 _____   5 _____

3 _____

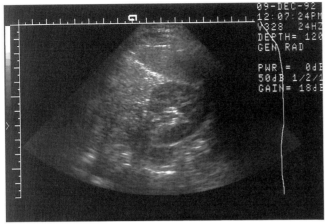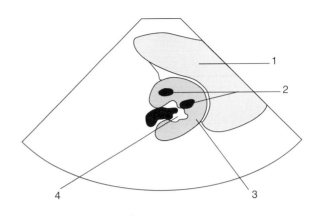

Figure 8–23. Transverse spleen and left kidney.

1 _____   3 _____

2 _____   4 _____

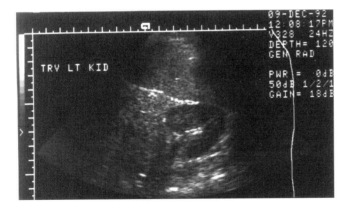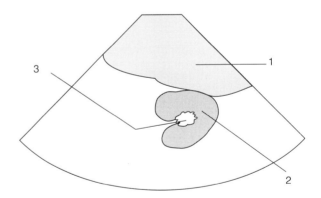

Figure 8–24. Transverse spleen and left kidney.

1 _____

2 _____

3 _____

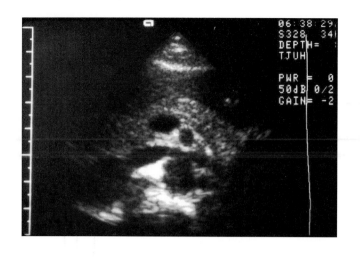
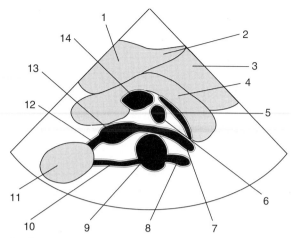

Figure 8–25. Transverse view of epigastric region.

1 _____		8 _____	
2 _____		9 _____	
3 _____		10 _____	
4 _____		11 _____	
5 _____		12 _____	
6 _____		13 _____	
7 _____		14 _____	

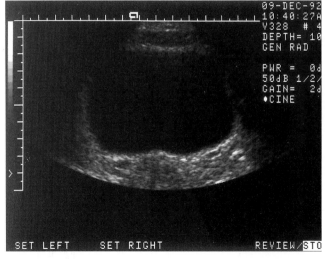
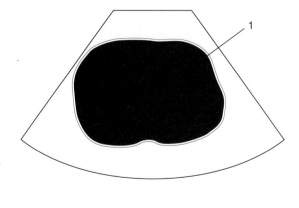

Figure 8–26. Urinary bladder.

1 _____

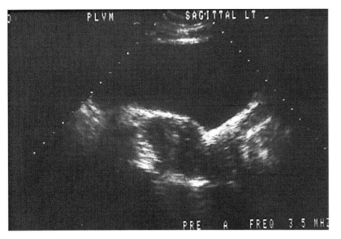 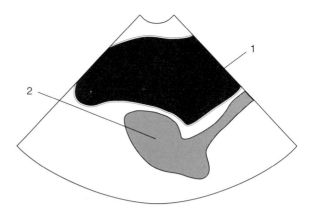

Figure 8–27. Urinary bladder.

1 _____   2 _____

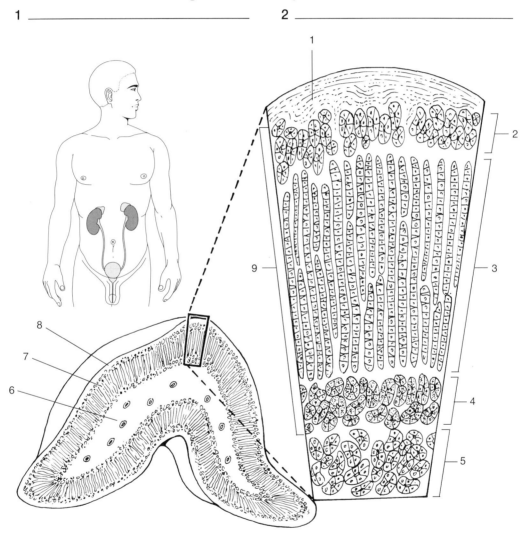

Figure 8–28. Adrenal gland.

1 _____   6 _____

2 _____   7 _____

3 _____   8 _____

4 _____   9 _____

5 _____

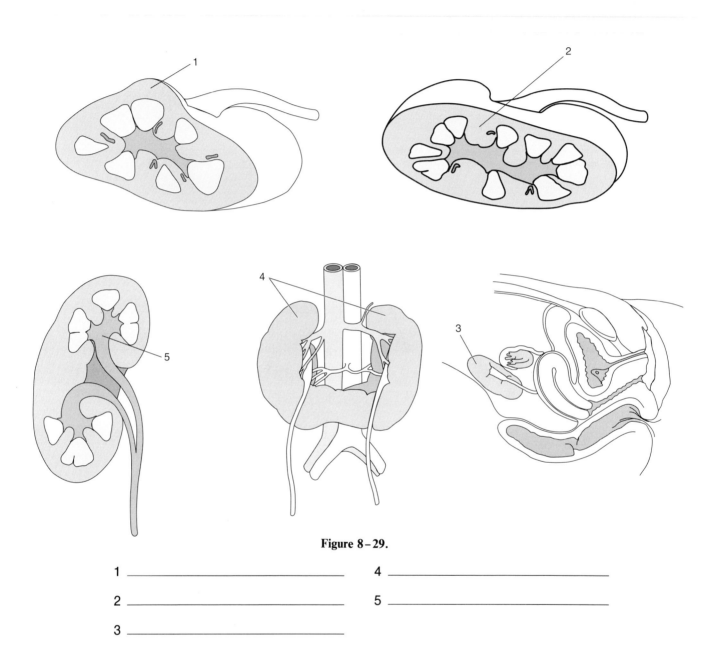

Figure 8–29.

1 _____   4 _____

2 _____   5 _____

3 _____

Chapter 9

THE SPLEEN

REVIEW QUESTIONS

1. Which of the following is not a reticuloendothelial function of the spleen?

   a. the storage of iron

   b. the production of lymphocytes

   c. the production of antibodies

   d. pitting function

2. The spleen arises from which embryological tissue?

   a. ectoderm

   b. mesoderm

   c. endoderm

3. The spleen begins to develop during the _____ week of gestation.

   a. fifth

   b. tenth

   c. fifteenth

   d. near term

4. Which function of the spleen ends shortly following birth?

   a. pitting function

   b. hematopoiesis

   c. culling function

   d. reservoir function

5. The upper limit of normal for the superior to inferior length of the spleen is _____ cm.

   a. 5–6

   b. 7–8

   c. 9–10

   d. 12–13

6. The spleen is essential to sustain life.

   a. true

   b. false

7. Which of the following describes a decrease in the number of platelets within the circulation?

   a. leukopenia

   b. hyalinization

   c. erythrocytosis

   d. thrombocytopenia

8. The spleen is a(n) _____ organ.

   a. retroperitoneal

   b. intraperitoneal

9. The cells within the spleen that perform the primary lymphocytic functions of the spleen are the

   a. red pulp

   b. white pulp

   c. malpighian corpuscles

   d. splenic sinuses

10. Phagocytosis of degenerating red blood cells occurs within which portion of the spleen?

   a. white pulp

   b. red pulp

   c. malpighian corpuscles

   d. splenic arteries

11. The spleen lies _____ to the tail of the pancreas.

a. anterior

b. inferior

c. medial

d. lateral

12. The left kidney lies _____ to the spleen.

a. anterior

b. posterior

c. superior

d. lateral

13. The most common splenic pigment is _____.

a. amyloid

b. anthrotic

c. malarial

d. hemosiderin

14. The malpighian corpuscles are found within which portion of the spleen?

a. splenic hilum

b. red pulp

c. white pulp

d. splenic cords

15. Which of the following statements best describes the sonographic appearance of the spleen?

a. a homogeneous organ with an echogenicity pattern similar to that of liver

b. a heterogeneous echo pattern

c. more echogenic than the pancreas

d. very echogenic due to its high volume of blood

16. Letter A on the following figure represents which correct orientation?

a. superior

b. inferior

c. anterior

d. lateral

A

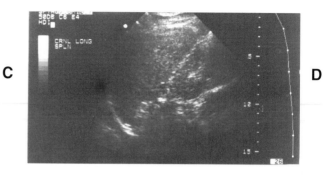

C

D

B

17. Letter C on the above figure represents which correct orientation?

a. superior

c. anterior

b. inferior

d. lateral

18. Letter D on the above figure represents which correct orientation?

a. superior

b. inferior

c. anterior

d. lateral

19. Letter A on the figure below represents which correct orientation?

a. superior

b. lateral

c. medial

d. posterior

20. Letter B on the figure below represents which correct orientation?

a. superior

c. medial

b. lateral

d. posterior

D

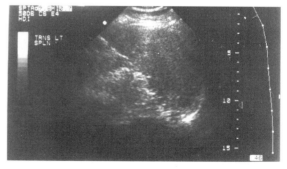

C

A

B

Identify the structures indicated in the following illustrations. These figures duplicate those found in **ULTRASONOGRAPHY: Introduction to Normal Structure and Functional Anatomy**. Refer to the textbook if you need help.

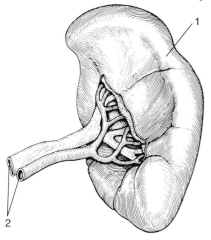

Figure 9–1. Splenic anatomy.

1 _____

2 _____

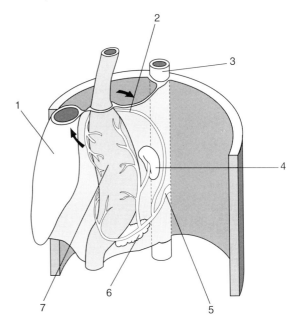

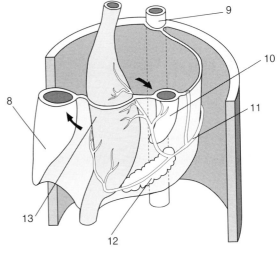

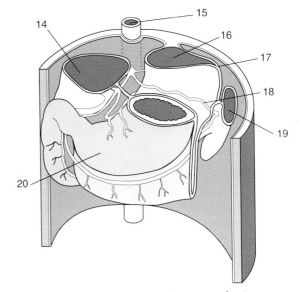

1 _____

2 _____

3 _____

4 _____

5 _____

6 _____

7 _____

8 _____

9 _____

10 _____

11 _____

12 _____

13 _____

14 _____

15 _____

16 _____

17 _____

18 _____

19 _____

20 _____

Figure 9–2. Prenatal development of spleen.

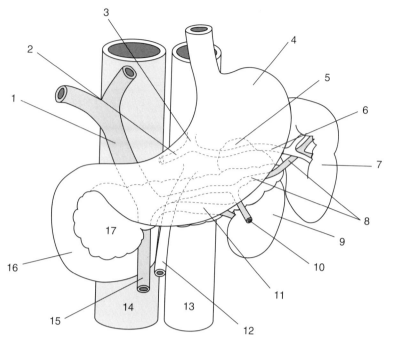

Figure 9–3. Spleen and surrounding anatomy.

1 _____

2 _____

3 _____

4 _____

5 _____

6 _____

7 _____

8 _____

9 _____

10 _____

11 _____

12 _____

13 _____

14 _____

15 _____

16 _____

17 _____

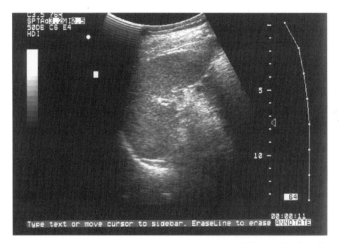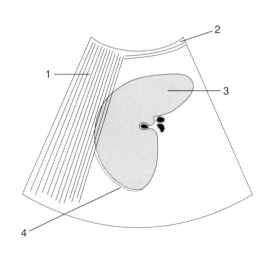

Figure 9–4. Coronal spleen.

1 _____   3 _____

2 _____   4 _____

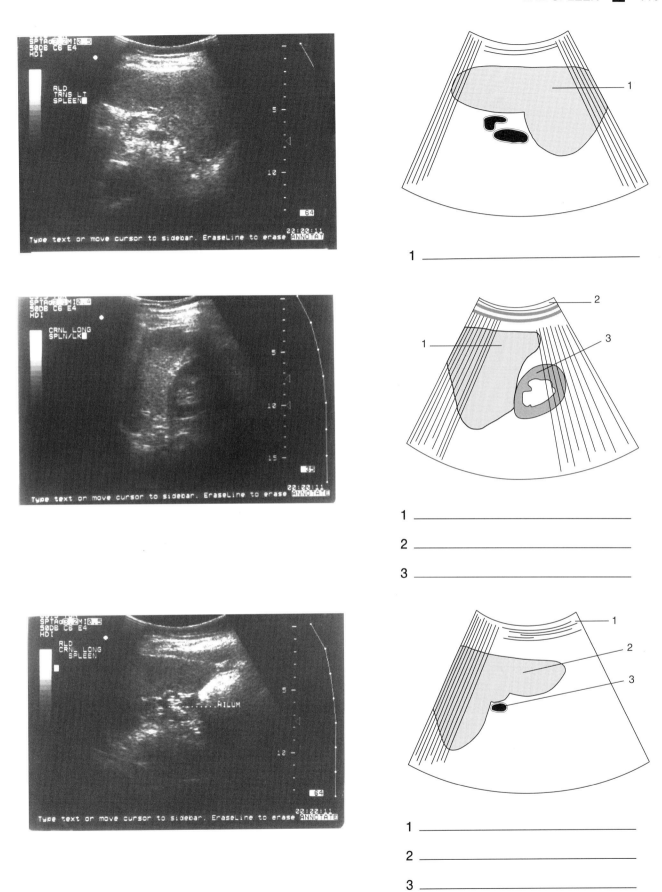

Figure 9-4. *Continued. Top*, Transverse spleen; *center*, Splenic/kidney interface; *bottom*, Coronal spleen.

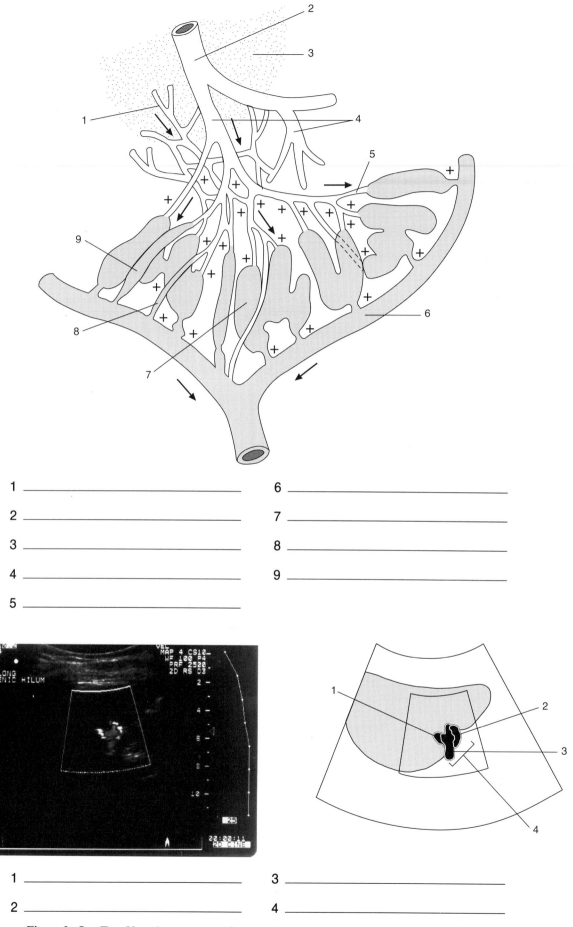

1 _____	6 _____
2 _____	7 _____
3 _____	8 _____
4 _____	9 _____
5 _____	

| 1 _____ | 3 _____ |
| 2 _____ | 4 _____ |

Figure 9–5. *Top*, Vascular anatomy of spleen; *bottom*, Color Doppler of splenic hilum.

Chapter 10

GASTROINTESTINAL SYSTEM
REVIEW QUESTIONS

1. The majority of the digestive processes of the GI tract take place in which portion of the tract?

a. mouth

b. stomach

c. small bowel

d. colon

2. Each of the following substances is digested and absorbed in the GI tract except

a. fats

b. proteins

c. carbohydrates

d. vitamins

e. water

f. there are no exceptions

Select the region that best approximates the location of each item.

3. _____ stomach	a. foregut
4. _____ proximal duodenum	b. midgut
5. _____ superior mesenteric	c. hindgut
6. _____ sigmoid	d. tailgut
7. _____ ascending colon	
8. _____ resorbed	
9. _____ celiac	
10. _____ inferior mesenteric	

11. The final position of the stomach is the result of

a. midgut

b. two rotations

c. division of the ventral mesentery

d. fixation of the mesenteric root

12. Midgut herniation out of and back into the abdominal cavity occurs during embryogenesis.

a. true

b. false

13. The terminal part of the esophagus connects with which portion of the stomach?

a. antrum

b. pylorus

c. fundus

d. cardiac

14. The stomach is located within each of the following regions except

a. left upper quadrant

b. left inguinal

c. epigastric

d. left hypochondrium

15. The stomach is separated from the pleura of the left lung and the apex of the heart by the

a. left hemidiaphragm

b. cardiac orifice

c. the left lobe of the liver

d. the falciform ligament

16. The posterior surface of the stomach is related to each of the following except the

a. diaphragm

b. superior pole of the left kidney

c. left lobe of the liver

d. anterior surface of the pancreas

e. gastric surface of the spleen

17. The stomach is located within the retro-peritoneum.

a. true

b. false

18. The small bowel is divided into three portions, including each of those shown below except

a. cecum

b. jejunum

c. duodenum

d. ileum

19. The duodenum contains portions located both in the peritoneal cavity and within the retroperitoneum.

a. true

b. false

20. The duodenal bulb is supported by the hepato-duodenal ligament and passes _____ to the common bile duct, the head of the pancreas, and the gastroduodenal artery.

a. medial

b. lateral

c. anterior

d. posterior

21. The portion of duodenum which receives the CBD via the ampulla of Vater is the

a. first (superior)

b. second (descending)

c. third (transverse)

d. fourth (ascending)

22. The large intestine begins in which of the following regions?

a. right hypochondrium

b. umbilical

c. left hypogastric

d. right inguinal

23. The ascending colon bends at the

a. splenic flexure

b. duodenojejunal flexure

c. hepatic flexure

d. ligament of Treitz

24. The smallest, widest, and most fixed portion of the small intestine is the

a. duodenum

b. ileum

c. ampulla of Vater

d. jejunum

25. The pylorus of the stomach is subdivided into three regions, including each of the following except

a. antrum

b. body

c. canal

d. sphincter

26. Which of the following is not a part of the large intestine?

a. appendix

b. cecum

c. rectum

d. ileum

e. right and left flexures

27. The colon is divided into segments called

a. rugae

b. alveoli

c. valvulae conniventes (valves of Kerckring)

d. haustra

28. The hormone which is released by the presence of fat in the intestine and which regulates gallbladder contraction and gastric emptying is

a. gastrin

b. secretin

c. cholecystokinin

d. lipase

29. After the major food products are mixed with digestive secretions and enzymes, carbohydrates are reduced to monosaccharides and disaccharides, proteins to amino acids and peptides, and fats to monoglycerides and fatty acids. These nutrients are then

a. absorbed through intestinal mucosa into the bloodstream

b. propelled into the duodenum for digestion

c. released into the large bowel for elimination

d. transported into the portal system via intestinal lymphatics

30. Visualization of the bowel is impeded by

a. fluid

b. air

c. gas

d. all of the above

e. b and c

31. The layers of the bowel wall create a characteristic sonographic appearance called a "gut signature." Up to _____ layers can be visualized.

a. three

b. four

c. five

d. six

32. The majority of the bowel wall layers recognizable on sonographic images are

a. anechoic

b. echogenic

c. hypoechoic

d. isoechoic

33. Each of the following may demonstrate a target appearance (bull's eye pattern) on sonographic images of the GI tract with the exception of

a. esophagogastric junction

b. inflamed appendix

c. stomach antrum

d. ileus

e. there are no exceptions

34. The ascending colon is anterolateral to the

a. tail of the pancreas

b. neck of the gallbladder

c. left iliac crest

d. lower pole of the right kidney

35. Abnormal bowel loops demonstrate peristalsis and are compressible, while normal loops are noncompressible.

a. true

b. false

Identify the structures indicated in the following illustrations. These figures duplicate those found in **ULTRASONOGRAPHY: Introduction to Normal Structure and Functional Anatomy**. Refer to the textbook if you need help.

1 _____

2 _____

3 _____

4 _____

5 _____

6 _____

7 _____

8 _____

9 _____

10 _____

11 _____

12 _____

13 _____

14 _____

15 _____

16 _____

17 _____

18 _____

19 _____

20 _____

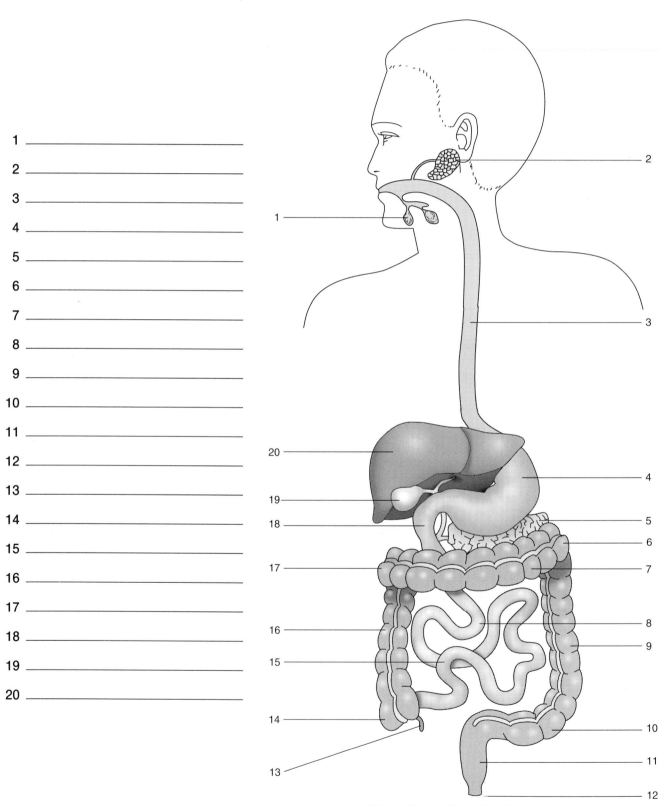

Figure 10-1. Gastrointestinal tract.

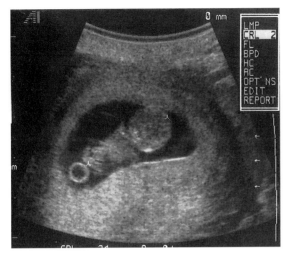 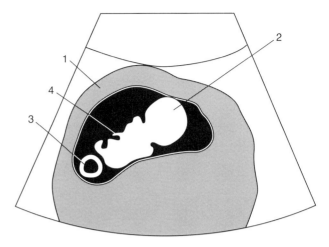

Figure 10-2. Fetal midgut herniation.

1 _____   3 _____

2 _____   4 _____

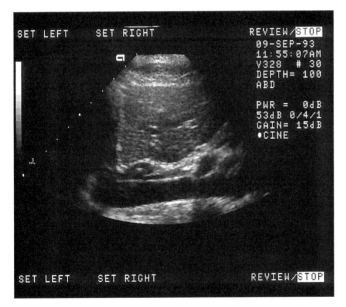 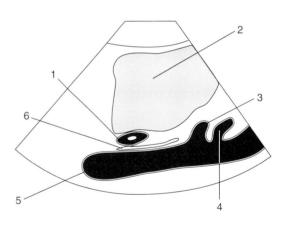

Figure 10-3. Longitudinal image esophagogastric junction.

1 _____   4 _____

2 _____   5 _____

3 _____   6 _____

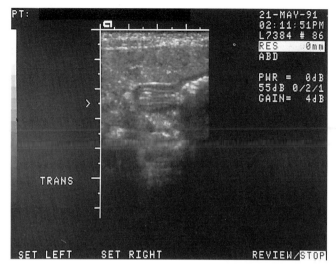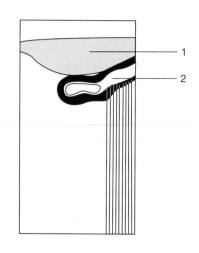

Figure 10–4. Transverse pylorus.

1 _____

2 _____

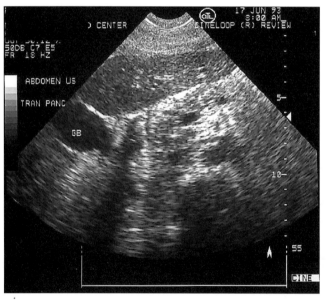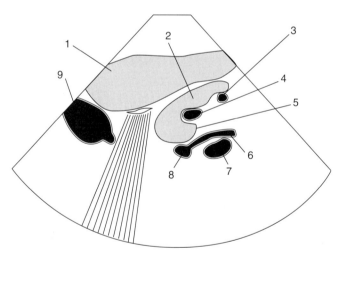

Figure 10–5. Transverse duodenum.

1 _____   6 _____

2 _____   7 _____

3 _____   8 _____

4 _____   9 _____

5 _____

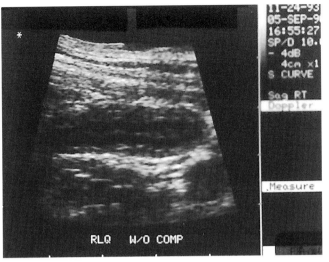
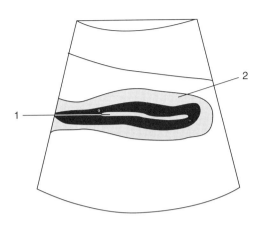

Figure 10-6. Normal appendix.

1 _____

2 _____

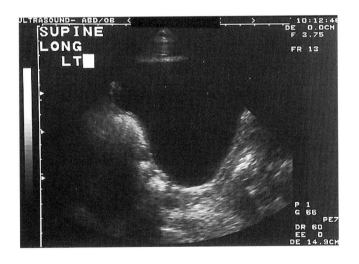
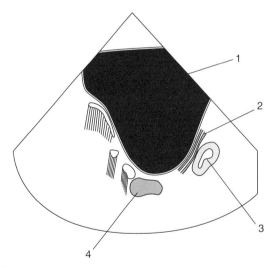

Figure 10-7. Longitudinal rectum.

1 _____ 3 _____

2 _____ 4 _____

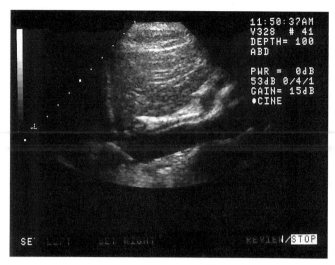
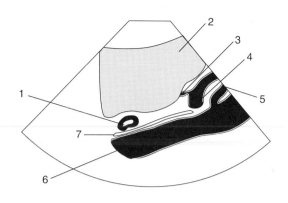

Figure 10-8. Longitudinal left gastric artery.

1 _____	5 _____
2 _____	6 _____
3 _____	7 _____
4 _____	

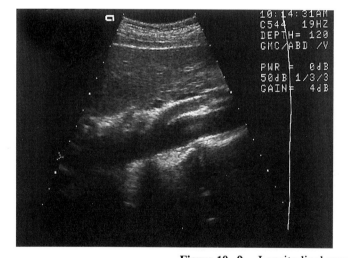
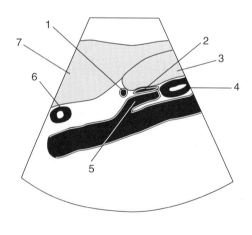

Figure 10-9. Longitudinal superior mesenteric artery.

1 _____	5 _____
2 _____	6 _____
3 _____	7 _____
4 _____	

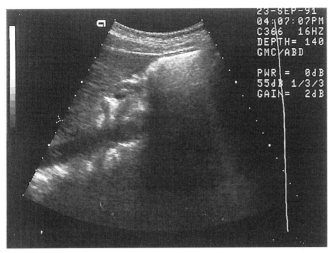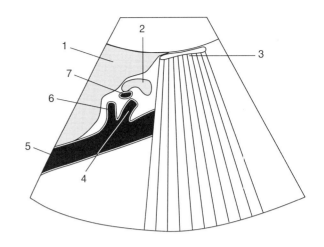

Figure 10–10. Longitudinal aorta.

1 _____   5 _____

2 _____   6 _____

3 _____   7 _____

4 _____

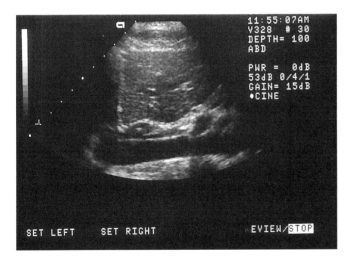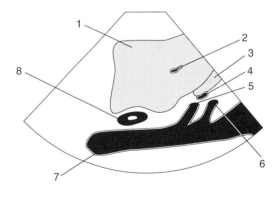

Figure 10–11. Longitudinal image esophagogastric junction.

1 _____   5 _____

2 _____   6 _____

3 _____   7 _____

4 _____   8 _____

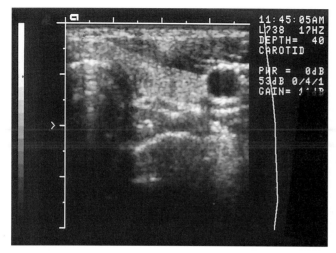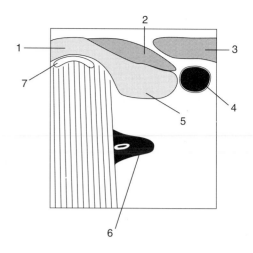

Figure 10-12. Transverse esophagus.

1 _____   5 _____

2 _____   6 _____

3 _____   7 _____

4 _____

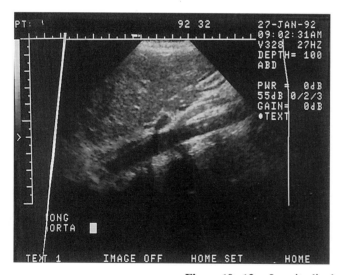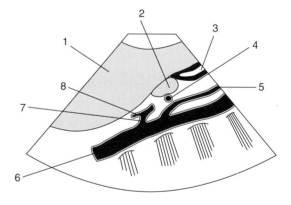

Figure 10-13. Longitudinal section stomach antrum.

1 _____   5 _____

2 _____   6 _____

3 _____   7 _____

4 _____   8 _____

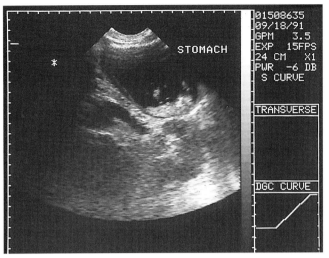
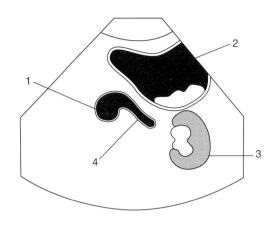

Figure 10–14. Transverse section stomach.

1 _____   3 _____

2 _____   4 _____

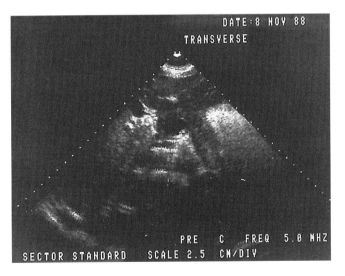
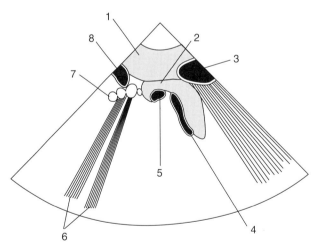

Figure 10–15. Transverse section duodenum.

1 _____   5 _____

2 _____   6 _____

3 _____   7 _____

4 _____   8 _____

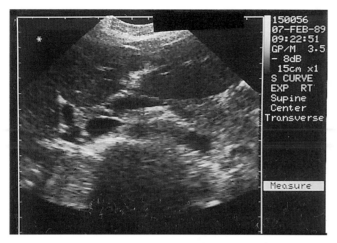 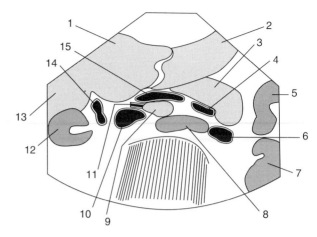

Figure 10–16. Transverse duodenojejunal flexure.

1 _____   9 _____

2 _____   10 _____

3 _____   11 _____

4 _____   12 _____

5 _____   13 _____

6 _____   14 _____

7 _____   15 _____

8 _____

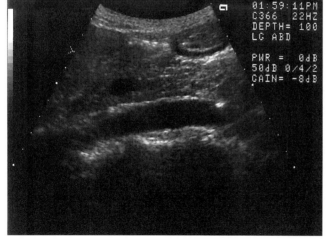 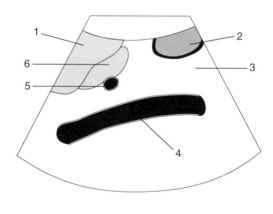

Figure 10–17. Compressed transverse colon.

1 _____   4 _____

2 _____   5 _____

3 _____   6 _____

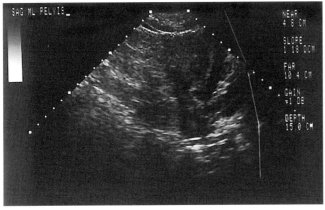 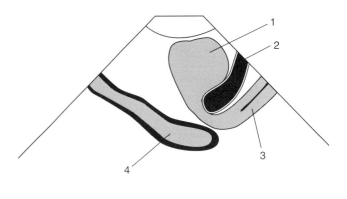

Figure 10–18. Sigmoid colon.

1 _____   3 _____

2 _____   4 _____

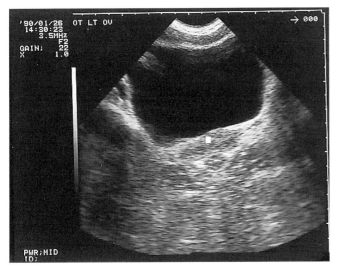 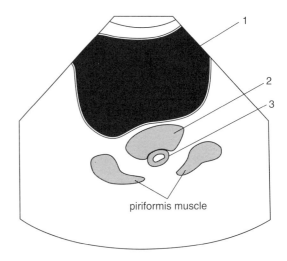

Figure 10–19. Transverse rectum.

1 _____

2 _____

3 _____

Chapter 11

REVIEW QUESTIONS

1. The normal aorta _____ in diameter as it progresses inferiorly.

a. increases

b. decreases

c. remains the same

d. turns into a vein

2. The common hepatic artery branches from the

a. proper hepatic artery

b. left hepatic artery

c. right hepatic artery

d. celiac axis

3. The normal aorta should not exceed _____ in diameter.

a. 3 cm

b. 4 cm

c. 2 cm

d. 1.5 cm

4. The abdominal aorta cannot be imaged in the _____ plane.

a. sagittal

b. transverse

c. longitudinal

d. thoracic

5. The celiac artery is a branch of the

a. aorta

b. iliac artery

c. gonadal artery

d. common hepatic artery

6. Arteriography is used to determine

a. arterial wall thickness

b. arterial stenosis

c. arterial flow rate

d. plethysmography

7. The inferior mesenteric artery is demonstrated with sonography

a. most of the time

b. none of the time

c. infrequently

d. consistently

8. The three branches of the celiac artery are

a. left gastric artery, splenic artery, common hepatic artery

b. left gastric artery, splenic artery, proper hepatic artery

c. right gastric artery, splenic artery, proper hepatic artery

d. right gastric artery, common and proper hepatic arteries

9. The structure(s) which receive(s) blood from the superior mesenteric artery include

a. brain

b. head and neck

c. intestines and pancreas

d. intestines and kidney

10. CT (compared with sonography) has the disadvantage of

a. being portable

b. producing radiation

c. being very inaccurate

d. utilizing magnetic waves to produce an image

Identify the structures indicated in the following illustrations. These figures duplicate those found in **ULTRASONOGRAPHY: Introduction to Normal Structure and Functional Anatomy**. Refer to the textbook if you need help.

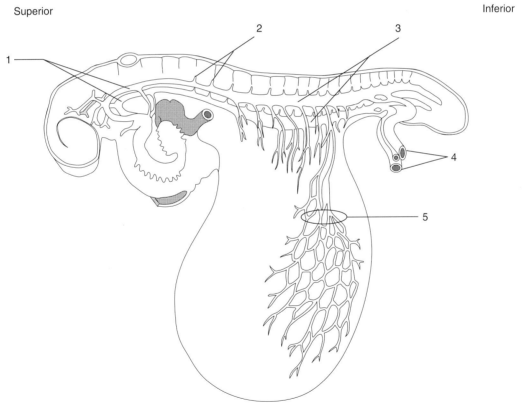

Superior   Inferior

Figure 11-1. Aortic embryologic development.

1 _____   4 _____

2 _____   5 _____

3 _____

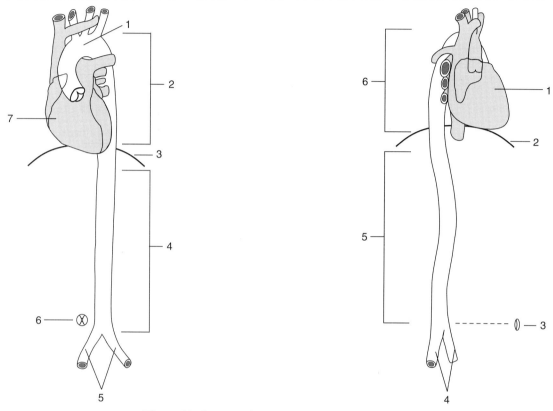

Figure 11–2. Anterior and lateral views of the aorta.

1 _____   1 _____

2 _____   2 _____

3 _____   3 _____

4 _____   4 _____

5 _____   5 _____

6 _____   6 _____

7 _____

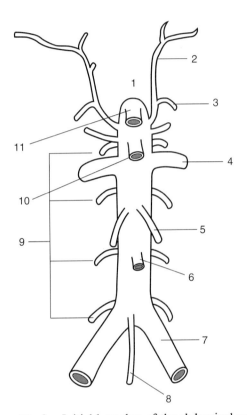

Figure 11-3. Initial branches of the abdominal aorta.

1 _____   7 _____

2 _____   8 _____

3 _____   9 _____

4 _____   10 _____

5 _____   11 _____

6 _____

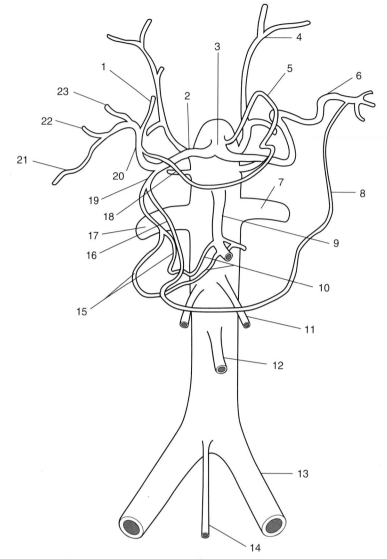

Figure 11–4. Branches of the abdominal aorta.

1 _____   13 _____

2 _____   14 _____

3 _____   15 _____

4 _____   16 _____

5 _____   17 _____

6 _____   18 _____

7 _____   19 _____

8 _____   20 _____

9 _____   21 _____

10 _____   22 _____

11 _____   23 _____

12 _____

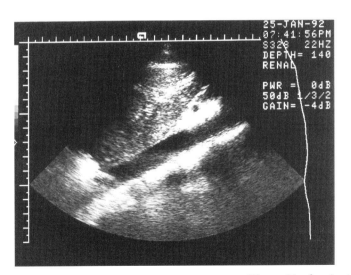

Figure 11-5. Cross-section of an arterial wall.

1 _____

2 _____

3 _____

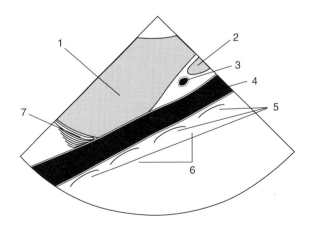

Figure 11-6. Aorta sagittal section.

1 _____ 5 _____

2 _____ 6 _____

3 _____ 7 _____

4 _____

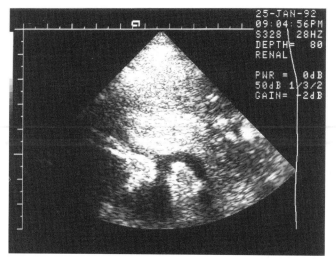
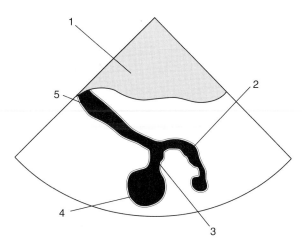

Figure 11–7. Aorta transverse section.

1 _____   4 _____

2 _____   5 _____

3 _____

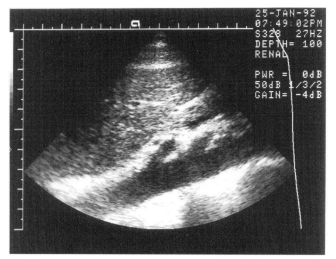
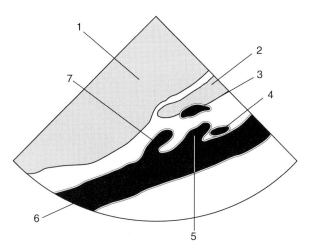

Figure 11–8. Aorta sagittal section.

1 _____   5 _____

2 _____   6 _____

3 _____   7 _____

4 _____

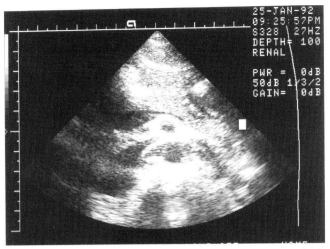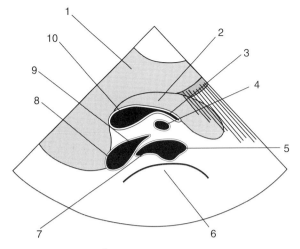

Figure 11–9. Abdominal vasculature transverse section.

1 _____   6 _____

2 _____   7 _____

3 _____   8 _____

4 _____   9 _____

5 _____   10 _____

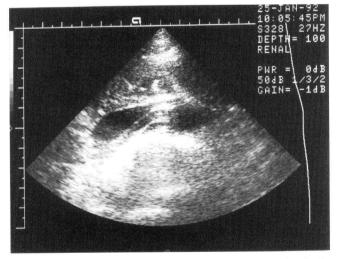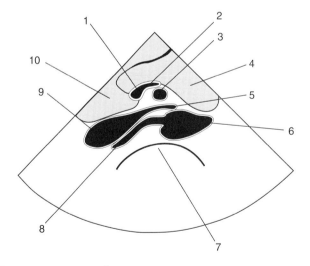

Figure 11–10. Abdominal vasculature transverse section.

1 _____   6 _____

2 _____   7 _____

3 _____   8 _____

4 _____   9 _____

5 _____   10 _____

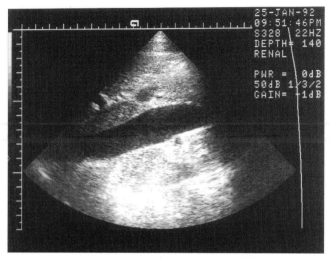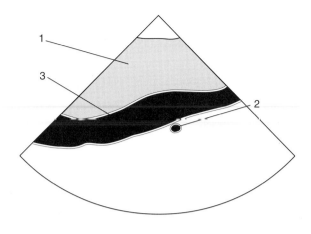

Figure 11–11. Inferior vena cava sagittal section.

1 _____

2 _____

3 _____

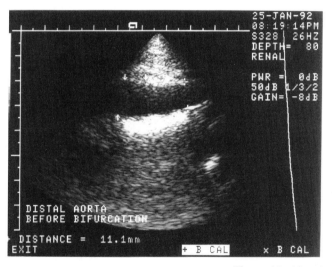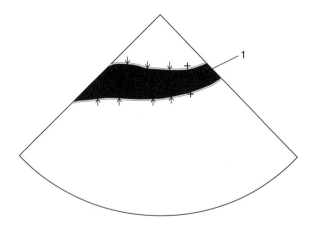

Figure 11–12. Aorta sagittal section.

1 _____

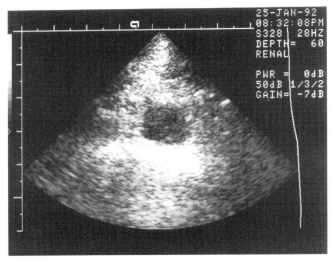 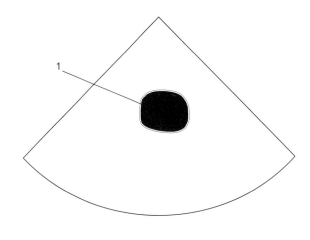

Figure 11–13. Aorta transverse section.

1 _____

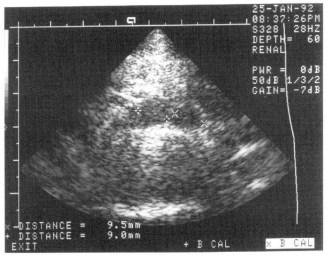 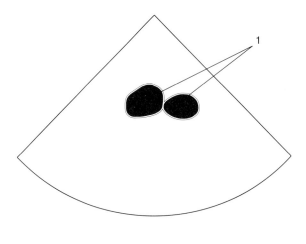

Figure 11–14. Iliac arteries transverse section.

1 _____

Chapter 12

REVIEW QUESTIONS

1. The normal venous system is a _____ pressure system.

a. low
b. high
c. medium
d. no

2. The left gonadal vein empties into the

a. inferior vena cava
b. right renal vein
c. left renal vein
d. right gonadal vein

3. The right gonadal vein empties into the

a. inferior vena cava
b. right renal vein
c. left renal vein
d. left gonadal vein

4. _____ is the gold standard when evaluating veins.

a. MRI
b. CT
c. venography
d. B-mode sonography

5. The superior mesenteric vein empties into the

a. inferior vena cava
b. portal vein
c. right renal vein
d. splenic vein

6. The primary function of the IVC is to

a. carry deoxygenated blood to the heart
b. carry deoxygenated blood from the heart
c. regulate heat dissipation from organs
d. act as a lymph drainage channel

7. Blood flow in veins should be _____ and _____

a. spontaneous and phasic
b. spontaneous and nonphasic
c. nonspontaneous and phasic
d. nonspontaneous and nonphasic

8. The inferior vena cava has a _____ tunica media than the aorta.

a. thicker
b. thinner
c. same size
d. more echogenic

9. The left renal vein has a(n) _____ course compared to the right renal vein.

a. longer
b. shorter
c. wider
d. identical

10. The lumen of all normal veins should appear without echoes except for

a. thrombus
b. valves and slow-moving blood
c. tumors
d. aggregated red blood cells

Identify the structures indicated in the following illustrations. These figures duplicate those found in **ULTRASONOGRAPHY: Introduction to Normal Structure and Functional Anatomy**. Refer to the textbook if you need help.

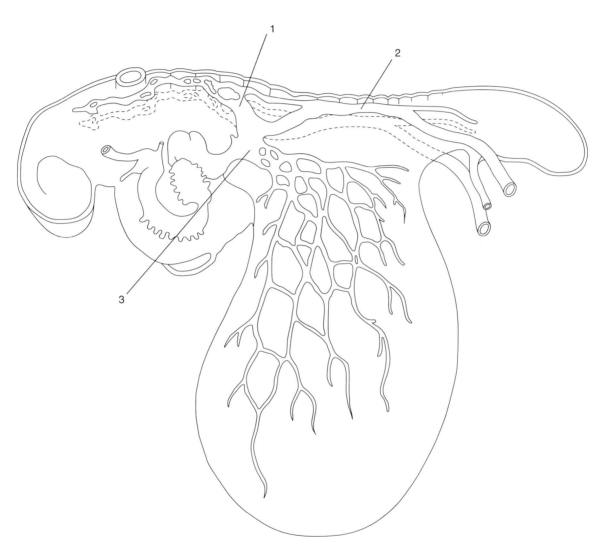

Figure 12–1. Inferior vena cava embryologic development.

1 _____

2 _____

3 _____

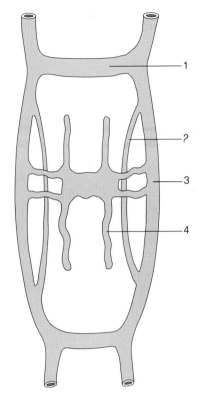

Figure 12-2. Anterior view cardinal venous system.

1 _____

2 _____

3 _____

4 _____

1 _____

2 _____

3 _____

4 _____

5 _____

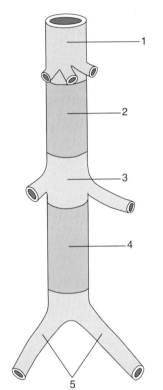

Figure 12-3. Inferior vena cava sections.

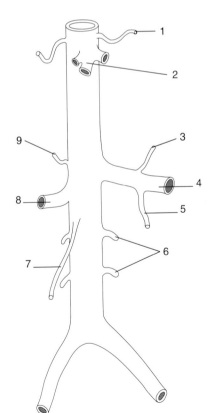

Figure 12-4. Inferior vena cava major tributaries.

1 _____

2 _____

3 _____

4 _____

5 _____

6 _____

7 _____

8 _____

9 _____

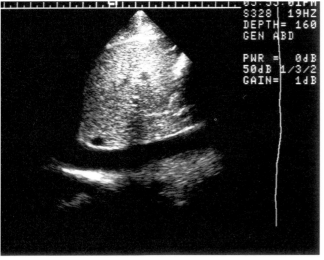
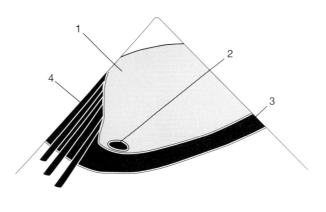

Figure 12–5. Inferior vena cava sagittal section.

1 _____   3 _____

2 _____   4 _____

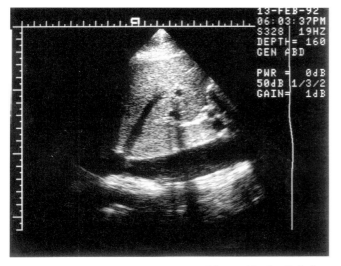
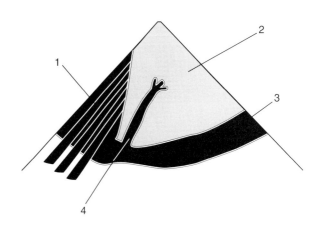

Figure 12–6. Inferior vena cava sagittal section.

1 _____   3 _____

2 _____   4 _____

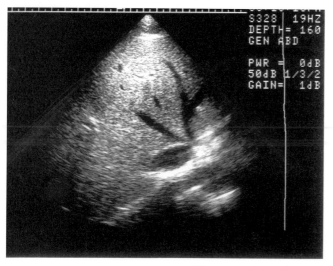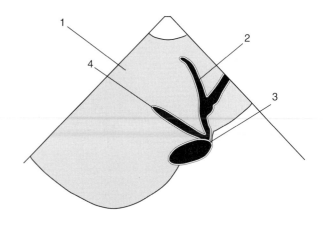

Figure 12-7. Inferior vena cava transverse section.

1 _____   3 _____

2 _____   4 _____

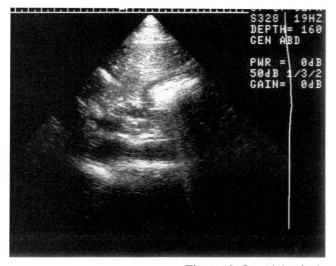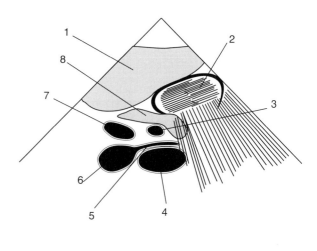

Figure 12-8. Abdominal vasculature transverse section.

1 _____   5 _____

2 _____   6 _____

3 _____   7 _____

4 _____   8 _____

Chapter 13

THE PORTAL VENOUS SYSTEM

REVIEW QUESTIONS

1. The portal vein supplies the liver with

a. arterial blood

b. venous blood

c. oxygenated blood

d. venous blood rich in nutrients

2. The portal vein empties blood from

a. the liver

b. the gastrointestinal system

c. the kidneys

d. the upper body trunk

3. The portal vein should

a. measure less than 13 mm

b. measure more than 13 mm

c. not be seen with sonography

d. be seen with sonography only when the patient is supine

4. The _____ and _____ join to form the portal vein.

a. superior mesenteric vein and splenic vein

b. inferior mesenteric vein and splenic vein

c. superior mesenteric vein and inferior mesenteric vein

d. inferior vena cava and superior mesenteric vein

5. The right portal vein branches into _____ and _____.

a. anterior and posterior

b. right and left

c. anterior and right

d. anterior and left

6. The superior mesenteric vein and inferior mesenteric vein empty the

a. liver

b. spleen

c. intestine

d. gallbladder

7. The portal veins are distinguished on a sonogram by their

a. highly echogenic walls

b. anechoic walls

c. echofree walls

d. bright red walls

8. The medial branch of the left portal vein feeds the

a. traditional left lobe of the liver

b. medial segment of the left lobe of the liver

c. right lobe of the liver

d. caudate lobe of the liver

9. The left main portal vein divides into _____ and _____.

a. anterior and posterior

b. right and left

c. right and anterior

d. anterior and left

10. Blood traveling from the spleen to the liver must pass through the

a. main portal vein

b. inferior mesenteric vein

c. superior mesenteric vein

d. portal artery

Identify the structures indicated in the following illustrations. These figures duplicate those found in **ULTRASONOGRAPHY: Introduction to Normal Structure and Functional Anatomy**. Refer to the textbook if you need help.

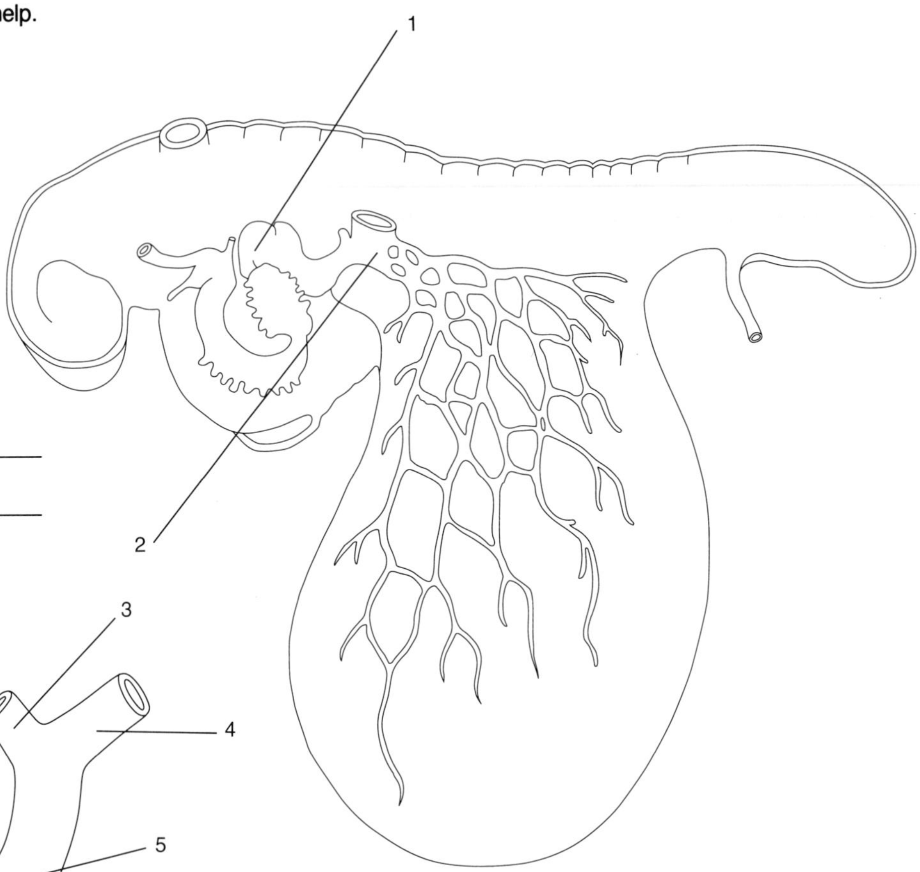

Figure 13-1. Portal vein embryologic development.

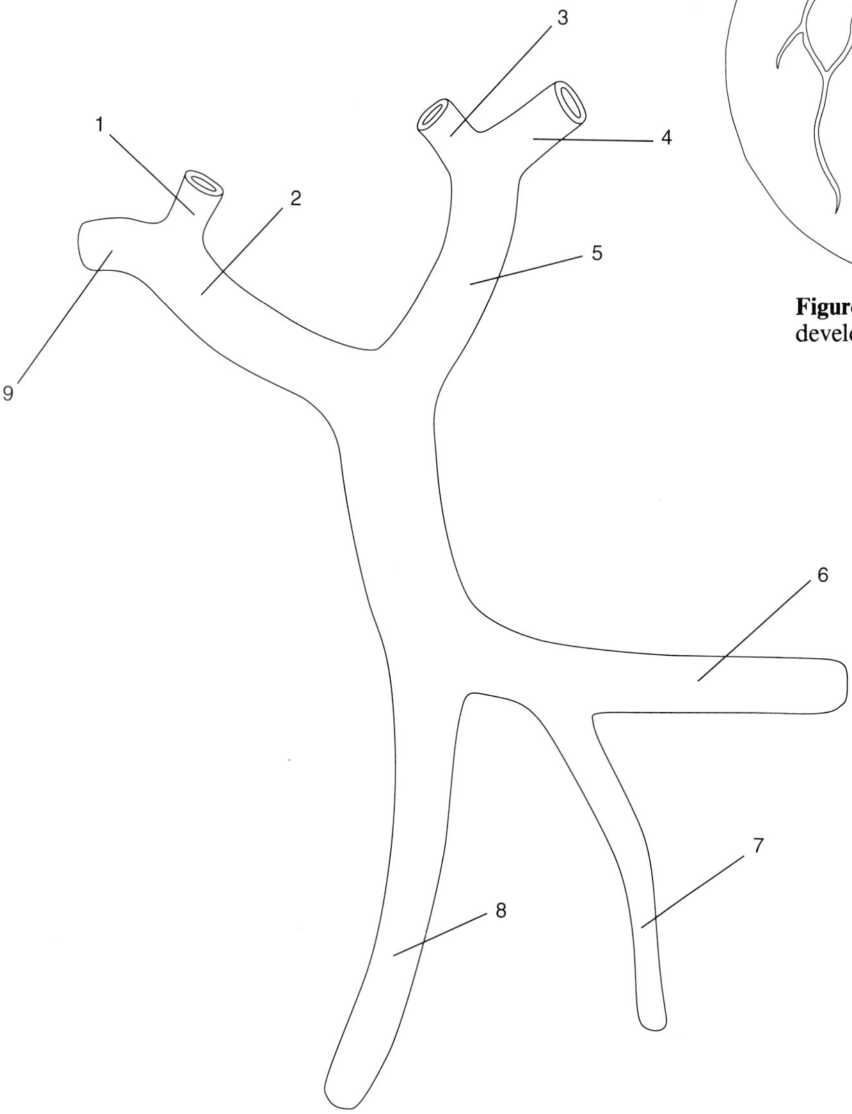

1 _____

2 _____

Figure 13-2. Portal venous system.

1 _____

2 _____

3 _____

4 _____

5 _____

6 _____

7 _____

8 _____

9 _____

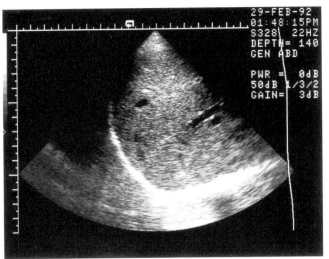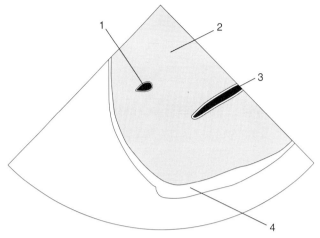

Figure 13–3. Liver vasculature sagittal section.

1 _____   3 _____

2 _____   4 _____

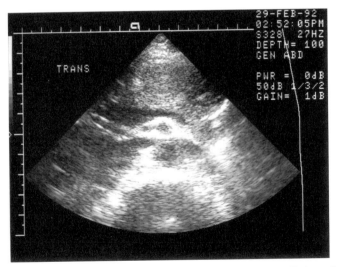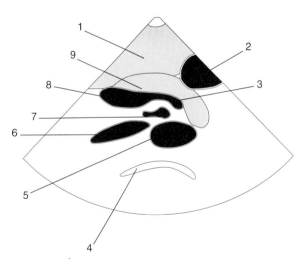

Figure 13–4. Epigastric transverse section.

1 _____   6 _____

2 _____   7 _____

3 _____   8 _____

4 _____   9 _____

5 _____

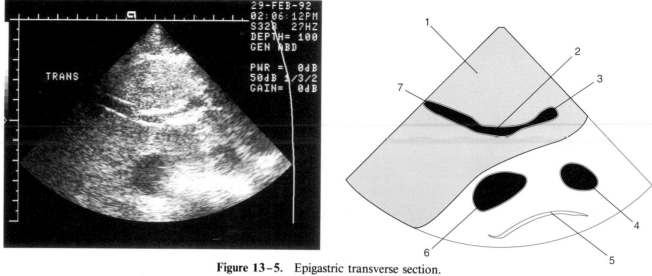

Figure 13-5. Epigastric transverse section.

1 _____   5 _____

2 _____   6 _____

3 _____   7 _____

4 _____

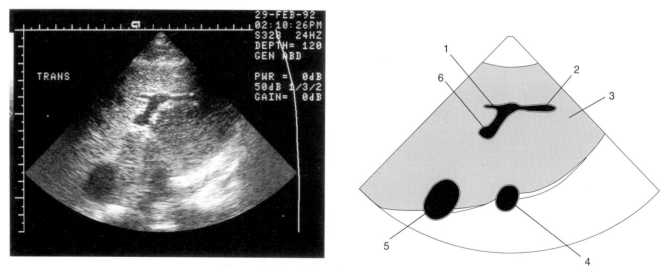

Figure 13-6. Epigastric transverse section.

1 _____   4 _____

2 _____   5 _____

3 _____   6 _____

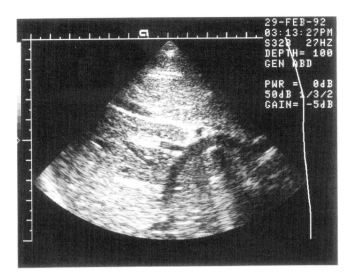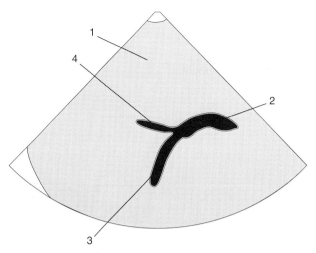

Figure 13–7. Right upper quadrant transverse section.

1 _____   3 _____

2 _____   4 _____

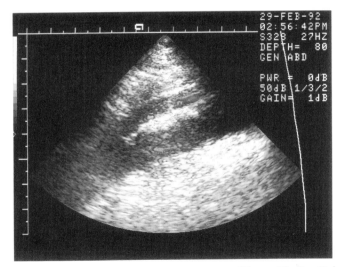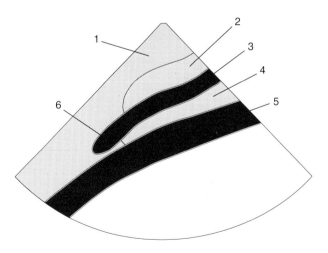

Figure 13–8. Epigastric sagittal section.

1 _____   4 _____

2 _____   5 _____

3 _____   6 _____

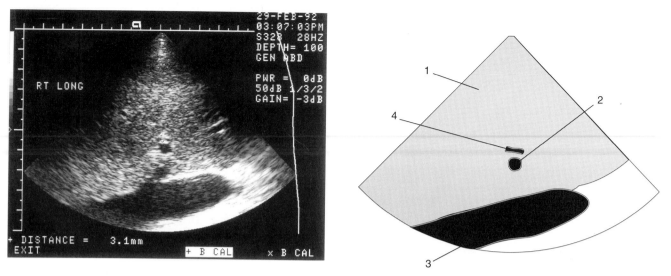

Figure 13–9. Right upper quadrant sagittal section.

1 _____   3 _____

2 _____   4 _____

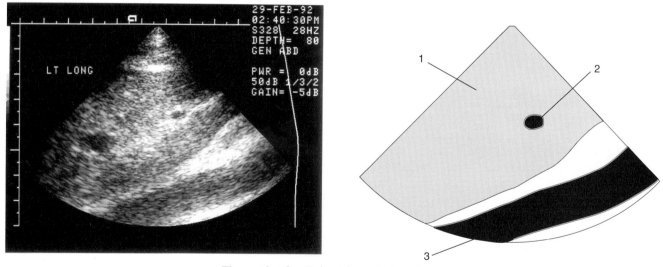

Figure 13–10. Epigastric sagittal section.

1 _____

2 _____

3 _____

Chapter 14

THE MALE PELVIS

REVIEW QUESTIONS

1. (T/F) Sex is determined by the presence or absence of the Y chromosome. The normal male fetus is identified as having the 46XY karyotype.

2. (T/F) The maximum diameter of the seminal vesicles is normally greater than 1 cm.

3. Which of the following is not found within each testis?

a. ductus epididymis

b. seminiferous tubules

c. rete testis

d. straight tubules

4. The left testicular vein drains into the

a. inferior vena cava

b. left internal iliac vein

c. right internal iliac vein

d. inferior mesenteric vein

e. left renal vein

5. Which of the following is not contained within the spermatic cord?

a. ductus deferens

b. pampiniform plexus

c. ejaculatory duct

d. cremaster muscle

6. (T/F) The peripheral zone is the largest zone of the glandular prostate.

7. (T/F) The penis is composed of three cylindrical masses of tissue: two corpora spongiosa and a single corpus cavernosum.

8. Which of the following is not visualized during an ultrasound examination of normal scrotum?

a. mediastinum testis

b. head of the epididymis

c. body of the epididymis

d. spermatic cord

9. (T/F) When scanning transrectally, the normal seminal vesicles will appear hyperechoic to the normal prostate gland.

10. The _____ zone is the only zone of the glandular prostate that can be individually differentiated on a transrectal ultrasound examination.

a. peripheral

b. central

c. transition

d. periurethral

Identify the structures indicated in the following illustrations. These figures duplicate those found in **ULTRASONOGRAPHY: Introduction to Normal Structure and Functional Anatomy**. Refer to the textbook if you need help.

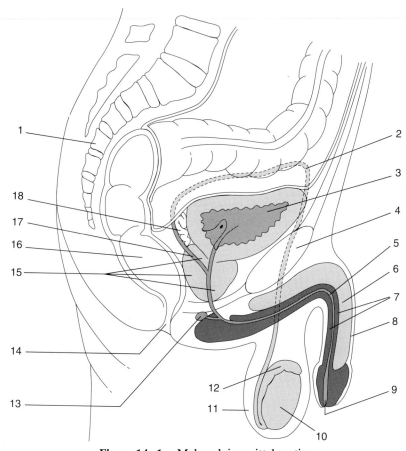

Figure 14–1. Male pelvis sagittal section.

1 _____	10 _____
2 _____	11 _____
3 _____	12 _____
4 _____	13 _____
5 _____	14 _____
6 _____	15 _____
7 _____	16 _____
8 _____	17 _____
9 _____	18 _____

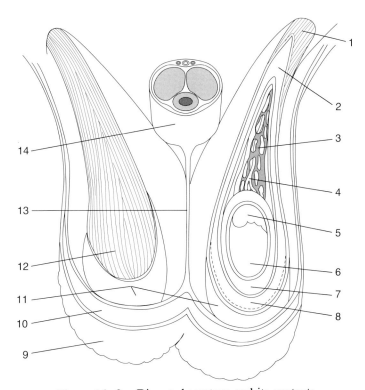

Figure 14–2. Dissected scrotum and its contents.

1 _____   8 _____

2 _____   9 _____

3 _____   10 _____

4 _____   11 _____

5 _____   12 _____

6 _____   13 _____

7 _____   14 _____

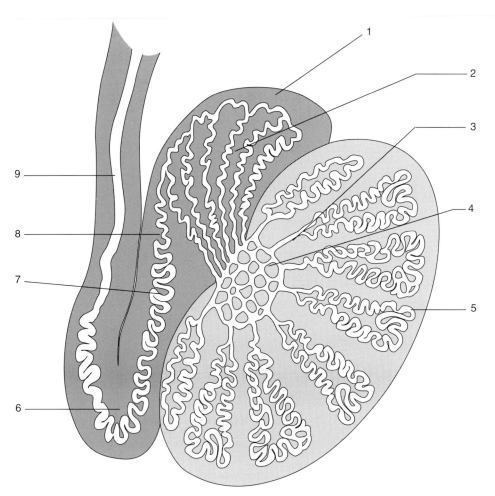

Figure 14-3. Enlarged sagittal section of testis, epididymis, and ductus (vas) deferens.

1 _____   6 _____

2 _____   7 _____

3 _____   8 _____

4 _____   9 _____

5 _____

CORONAL PLANE

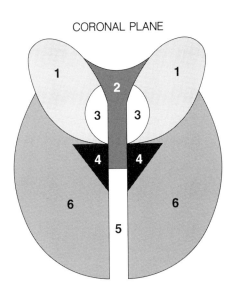

SAGITTAL PLANE

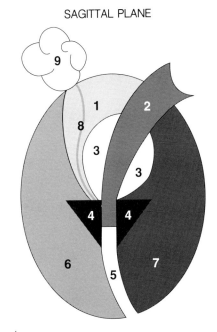

Figure 14–4. Prostate zonal anatomy.

1 _____

2 _____

3 _____

4 _____

5 _____

6 _____

7 _____

8 _____

9 _____

1 _____

2 _____

3 _____

4 _____

5 _____

6 _____

7 _____

8 _____

9 _____

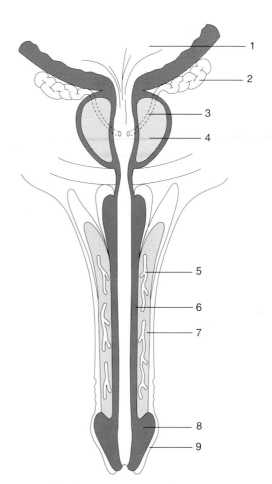

Penis anatomy coronal plane.

1 _____

2 _____

3 _____

4 _____

5 _____

6 _____

7 _____

8 _____

9 _____

10 _____

11 _____

12 _____

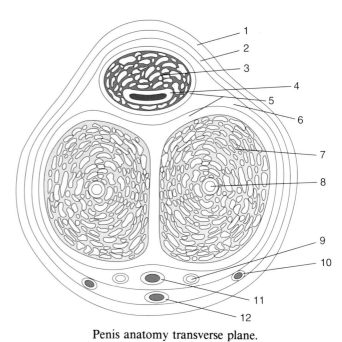

Penis anatomy transverse plane.

Figure 14–5.

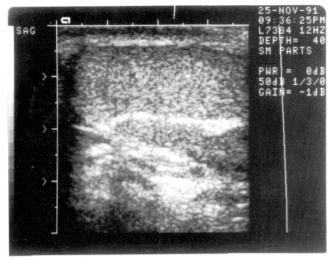
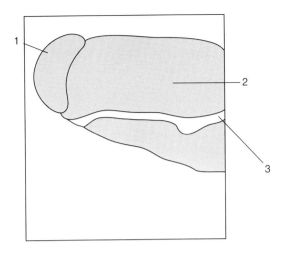

Figure 14-6. Testis sagittal section.

1 _____

2 _____

3 _____

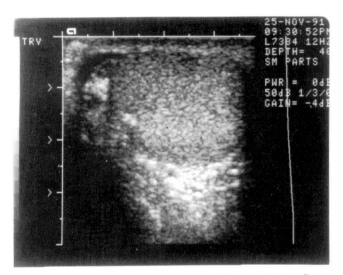
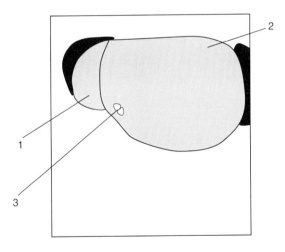

Figure 14-7. Scrotum transverse section.

1 _____

2 _____

3 _____

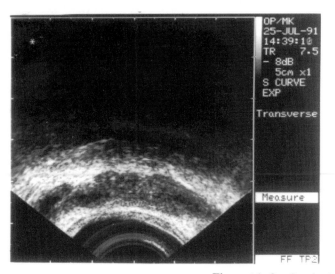
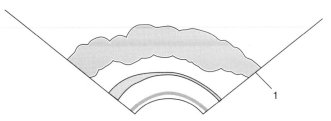

Figure 14-8. Seminal vesicles transverse section.

1 _____

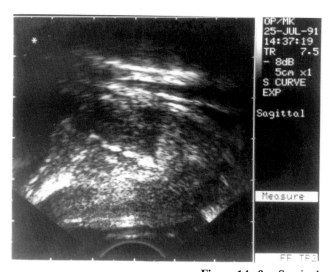
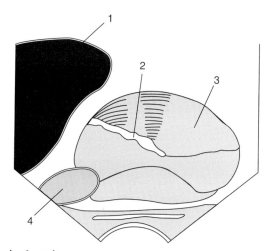

Figure 14-9. Seminal vesicle sagittal section.

1 _____   3 _____

2 _____   4 _____

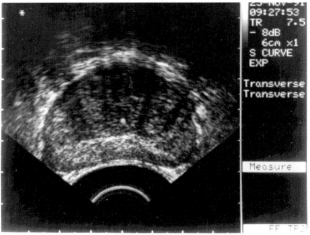
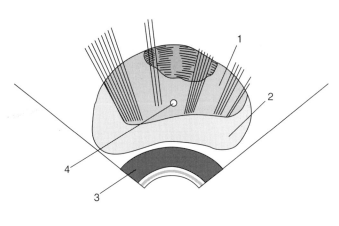

Figure 14-10. Prostate transverse section.

1 _____   3 _____

2 _____   4 _____

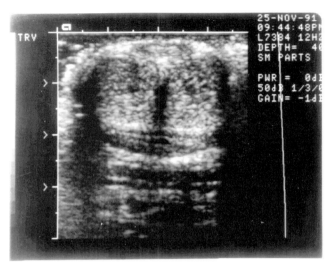
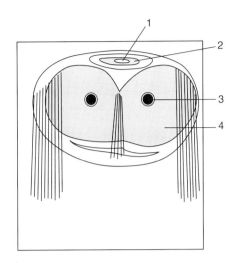

Figure 14–11. Penis transverse section.

1 _____   3 _____

2 _____   4 _____

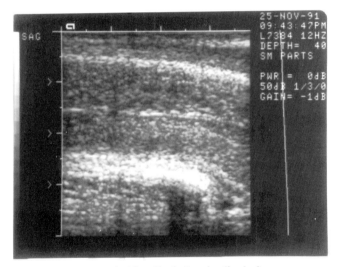
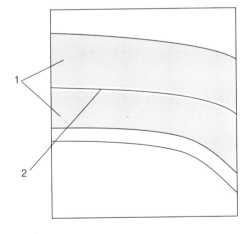

Figure 14–12. Penis longitudinal view.

1 _____

2 _____

Chapter 15

REVIEW QUESTIONS

1. Which of the following statements most accurately describes the anatomic relationships among the ovary, the ureter, and the internal iliac vessels?

   a. the ureter is posterior to the ovary, while the internal iliac vessels are anterior to the ovary

   b. the ureter is anterior to the ovary, while the internal iliac vessels are posterior to the ovary

   c. the ureter and internal iliac vessels both lie posterior to the ovary

   d. the ureter and internal iliac vessels both lie anterior to the ovary

2. Which of the following is used to divide the pelvic cavity into the pelvis major (false pelvis) and the pelvis minor (true pelvis)?

   a. pubic symphysis

   b. linea alba

   c. linea terminalis

   d. iliac crests

3. Which of the following muscles *do not* lie within the true pelvis?

   a. iliacus muscles

   b. piriformis muscles

   c. levator ani muscles

   d. obturator internus muscles

4. In which structure(s) are the hormones estrogen and progesterone produced in the female body?

   a. anterior pituitary gland

   b. ovarian medulla

   c. ovarian follicles

   d. uterine endometrium

5. The fibrous tissue mass remaining in the ovarian cortex following ovulation and the regression of the corpus luteum is called

   a. corpus albicans

   b. graafian follicle

   c. linea alba

   d. granulosa luteal cells

6. The arteries within the uterus which penetrate the myometrium are the

   a. spiral arteries

   b. arcuate arteries

   c. straight arteries

   d. radial arteries

7. The region of the *uterus* where the fallopian tube passes through the uterine wall and communicates with the uterine cavity is called the

   a. corpus

   b. cornu

   c. fundus

   d. infundibulum

8. Which of the following is the *outermost* layer of the ovary?

   a. tunica externa

   b. tunica albuginea

   c. visceral peritoneum

   d. germinal epithelium

9. Which of the following support structures anchors the ovary loosely to the uterine cornu?

   a. mesovarium

   b. ovarian ligament

   c. round ligament

   d. cardinal ligament

   e. infundibulopelvic ligament

10. Which of the following support structures extends from the uterine cornu, passes over the pelvic brim, through the inguinal canal, and is secured at the labia majora?

    a. round ligament

    b. broad ligament

    c. cardinal ligament

    d. uterosacral ligament

11. The most echogenic layer of the vagina is the

    a. vaginal mucosa

    b. muscular wall

    c. vaginal canal

    d. vaginal serosa

12. Bicornuate uterus is a congenital malformation caused by incomplete fusion of which structures during embryogenesis?

    a. wolffian ducts

    b. müllerian ducts

    c. urogenital sinuses

    d. mesonephros

13. On ultrasound, the skeletal muscles of the abdomen and pelvis appear _____ compared to their surrounding structures.

    a. hyperechoic

    b. hypoechoic

    c. isoechoic

    d. anechoic

14. The space between the pubic symphysis and the anterior wall of the urinary bladder is called the

    a. anterior cul de sac

    b. vesicouterine pouch

    c. uterovesical junction

    d. space of Retzius

15. Name the gonadotropin responsible for maintaining the corpus luteum.

    a. follicle stimulating hormone

    b. estrogen

    c. progesterone

    d. luteinizing hormone

Identify the structures indicated in the following illustrations. These figures duplicate those found in **ULTRASONOGRAPHY: Introduction to Normal Structure and Functional Anatomy**. Refer to the textbook if you need help.

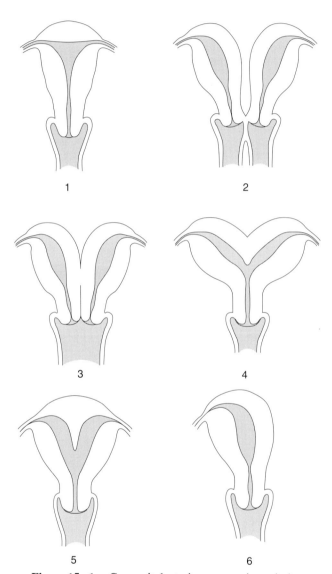

Figure 15–1. Congenital uterine anatomic variations.

1 _____   4 _____

2 _____   5 _____

3 _____   6 _____

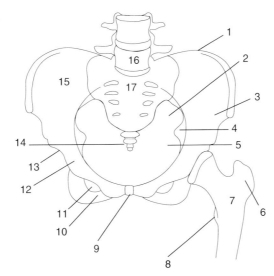

Figure 15-2. The pelvic skeleton.

1 _____   10 _____

2 _____   11 _____

3 _____   12 _____

4 _____   13 _____

5 _____   14 _____

6 _____   15 _____

7 _____   16 _____

8 _____   17 _____

9 _____

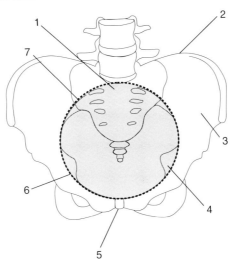

Figure 15-3. The true and false pelvis.

1 _____   5 _____

2 _____   6 _____

3 _____   7 _____

4 _____

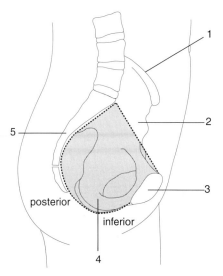

Figure 15–4. The true pelvis.

1 _____   4 _____

2 _____   5 _____

3 _____

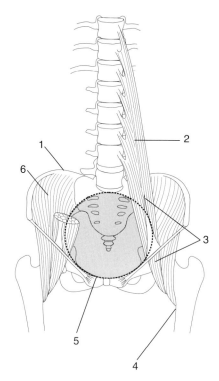

Figure 15–5. Muscles of the false pelvis.

1 _____   4 _____

2 _____   5 _____

3 _____   6 _____

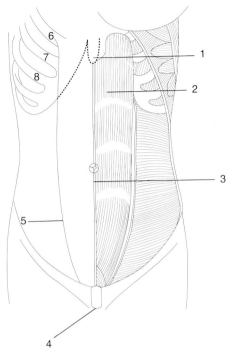

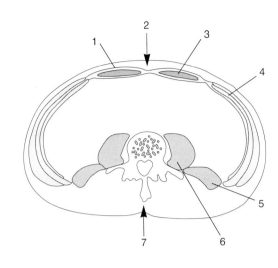

Figure 15-6. Abdominopelvic cavity skeletal muscles.

1 _____

2 _____

3 _____

4 _____

5 _____

6 _____

7 _____

1 _____

2 _____

3 _____

4 _____

5 _____

6 _____

7 _____

8 _____

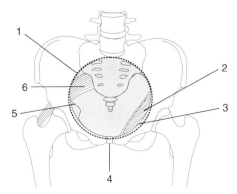

Figure 15-7. Muscles of the true pelvis.

1 _____   4 _____

2 _____   5 _____

3 _____   6 _____

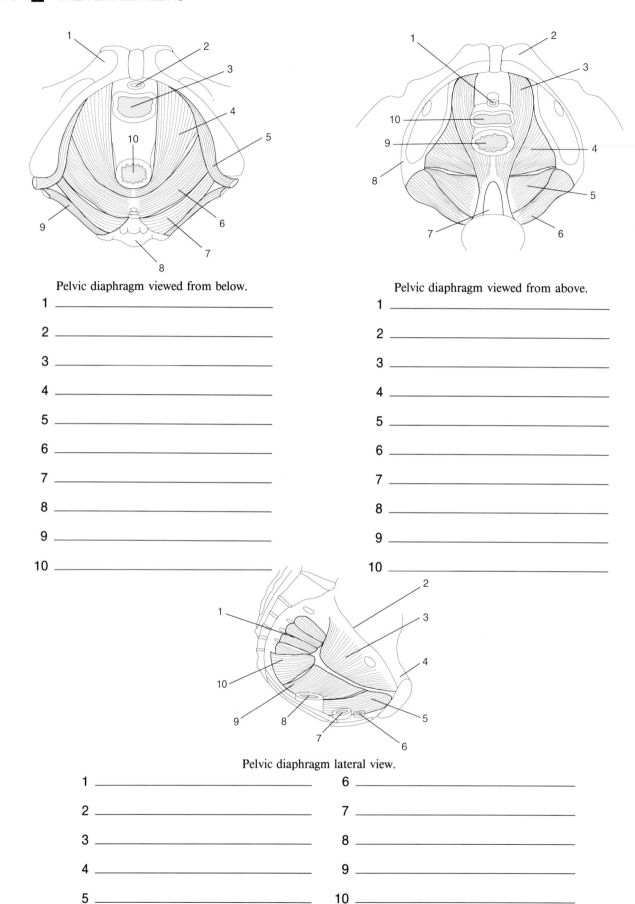

Pelvic diaphragm viewed from below.

1 _____
2 _____
3 _____
4 _____
5 _____
6 _____
7 _____
8 _____
9 _____
10 _____

Pelvic diaphragm viewed from above.

1 _____
2 _____
3 _____
4 _____
5 _____
6 _____
7 _____
8 _____
9 _____
10 _____

Pelvic diaphragm lateral view.

1 _____   6 _____
2 _____   7 _____
3 _____   8 _____
4 _____   9 _____
5 _____   10 _____

Figure 15–8.

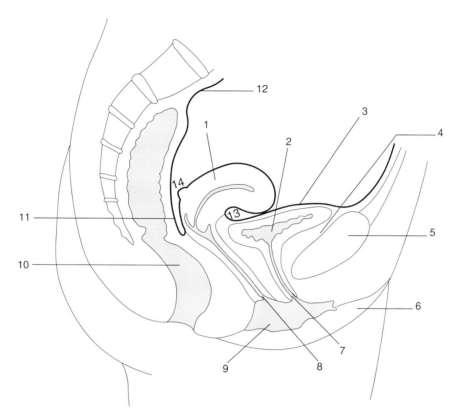

Figure 15–9. Female pelvis sagittal section.

1 _____   8 _____

2 _____   9 _____

3 _____   10 _____

4 _____   11 _____

5 _____   12 _____

6 _____   13 _____

7 _____   14 _____

1 _____

2 _____

3 _____

4 _____

5 _____

6 _____

7 _____

8 _____

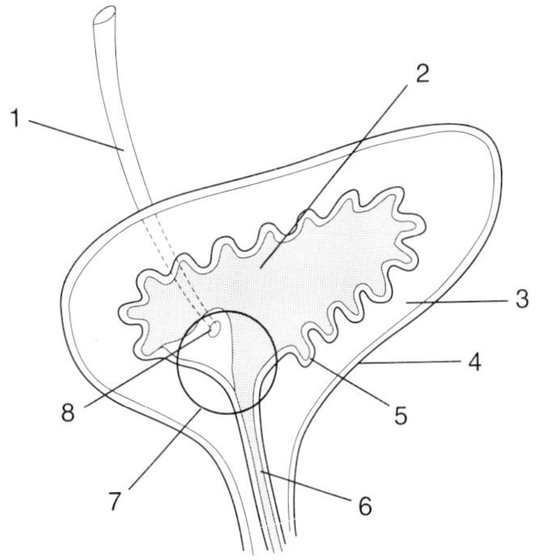

Figure 15–10. Urinary bladder.

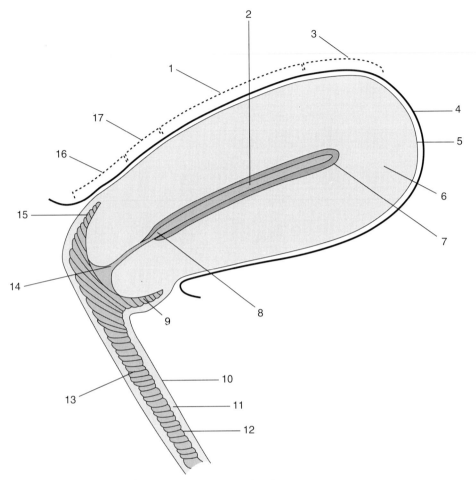

Figure 15–11. The vagina and uterus.

1 _____	10 _____
2 _____	11 _____
3 _____	12 _____
4 _____	13 _____
5 _____	14 _____
6 _____	15 _____
7 _____	16 _____
8 _____	17 _____
9 _____	

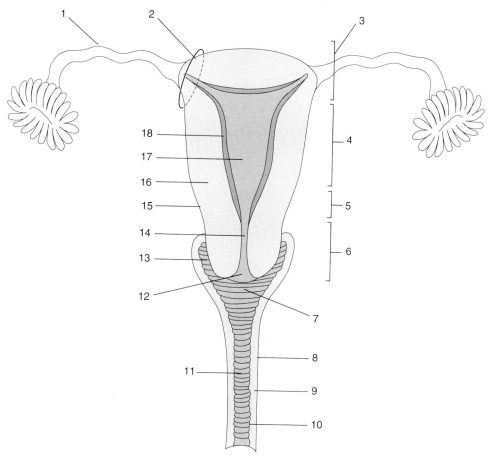

Figure 15–12. Genital tract coronal section.

1 _____   10 _____

2 _____   11 _____

3 _____   12 _____

4 _____   13 _____

5 _____   14 _____

6 _____   15 _____

7 _____   16 _____

8 _____   17 _____

9 _____   18 _____

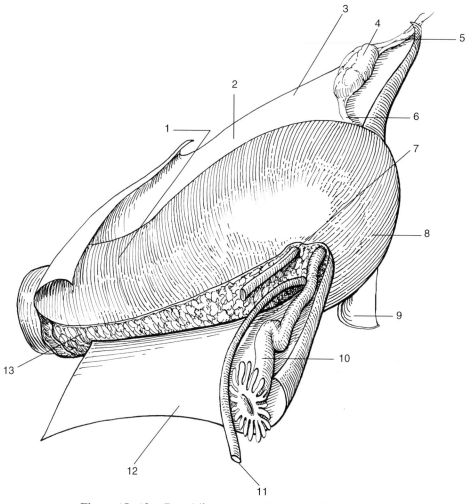

Figure 15-13. Broad ligaments and surrounding structures.

1 _____	8 _____
2 _____	9 _____
3 _____	10 _____
4 _____	11 _____
5 _____	12 _____
6 _____	13 _____
7 _____	

Left

Right

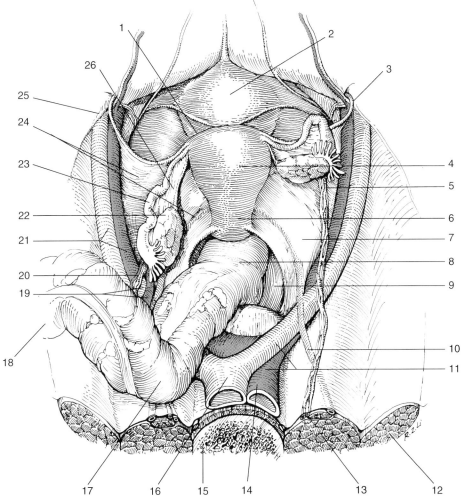

Figure 15–14. Pelvic ligaments and surrounding structures.

1 _____	14 _____
2 _____	15 _____
3 _____	16 _____
4 _____	17 _____
5 _____	18 _____
6 _____	19 _____
7 _____	20 _____
8 _____	21 _____
9 _____	22 _____
10 _____	23 _____
11 _____	24 _____
12 _____	25 _____
13 _____	26 _____

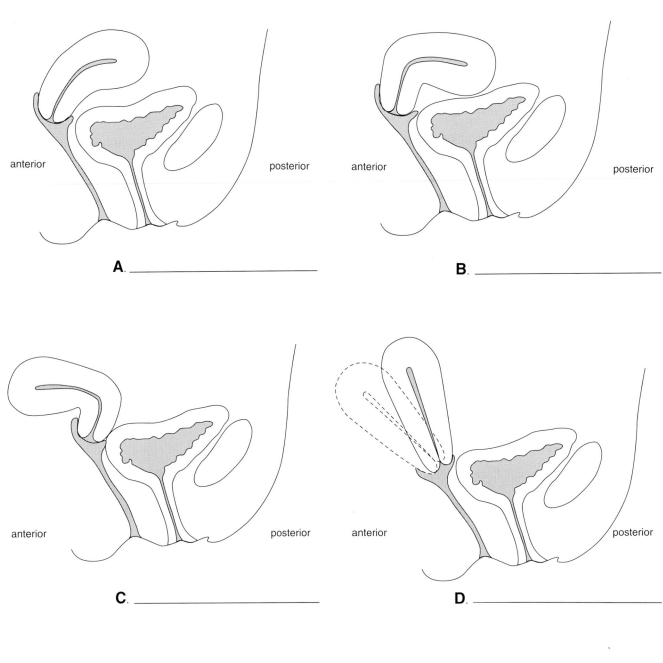

A. _____

B. _____

C. _____

D. _____

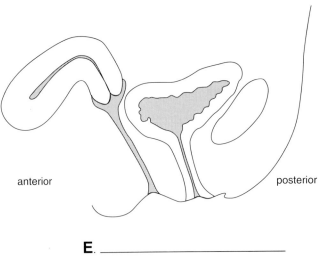

E. _____

Figure 15–15. Variations in uterine positions.

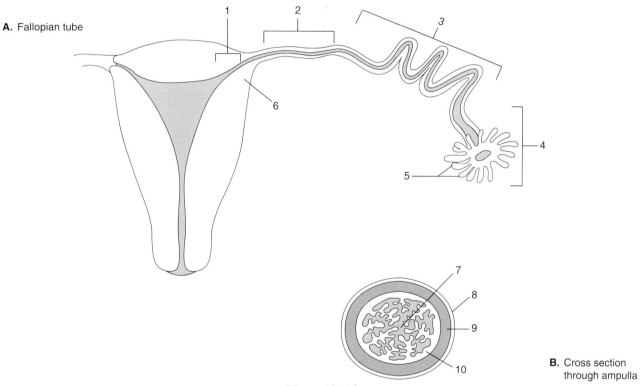

A. Fallopian tube

B. Cross section through ampulla

Figure 15–16.

1 _____   6 _____

2 _____   7 _____

3 _____   8 _____

4 _____   9 _____

5 _____   10 _____

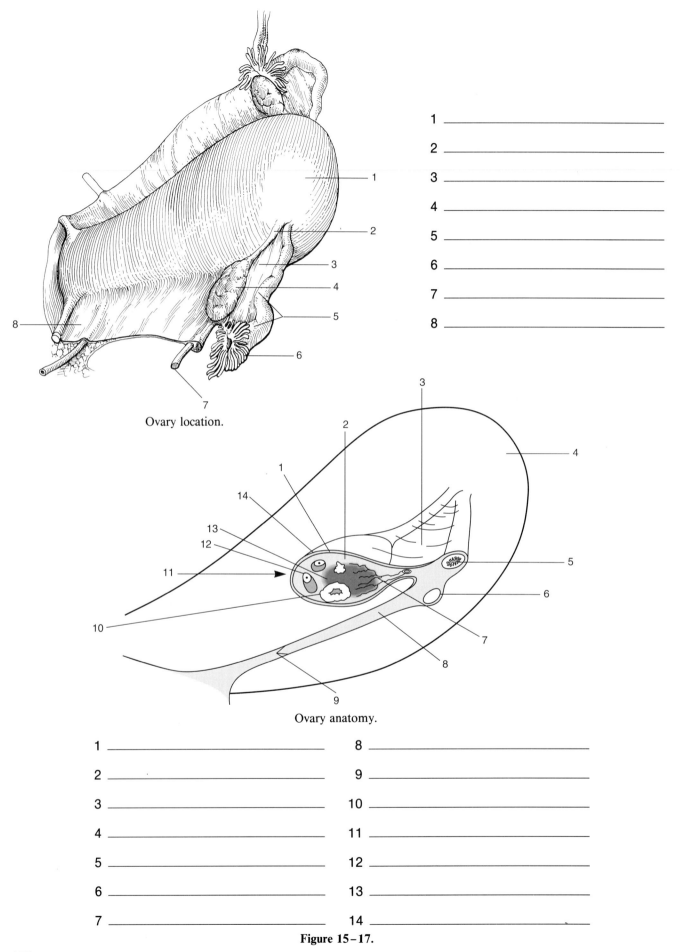

Ovary location.

Ovary anatomy.

1 _____
2 _____
3 _____
4 _____
5 _____
6 _____
7 _____
8 _____

1 _____   8 _____
2 _____   9 _____
3 _____   10 _____
4 _____   11 _____
5 _____   12 _____
6 _____   13 _____
7 _____   14 _____

Figure 15–17.

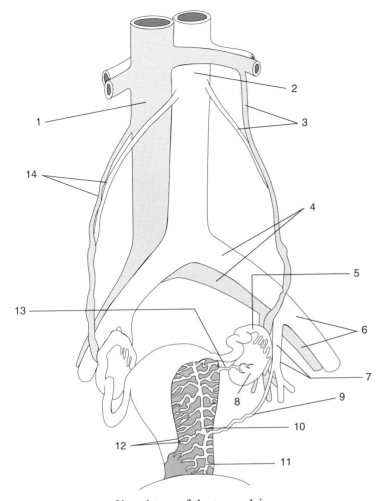

Vasculature of the true pelvis.

1 _____

2 _____

3 _____

4 _____

5 _____

6 _____

7 _____

8 _____

9 _____

10 _____

11 _____

12 _____

13 _____

14 _____

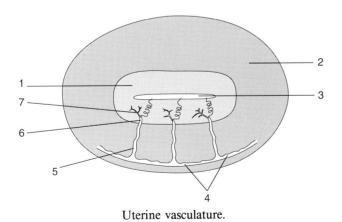

Uterine vasculature.

1 _____

2 _____

3 _____

4 _____

5 _____

6 _____

7 _____

Figure 15–18.

DISPLAY MONITOR

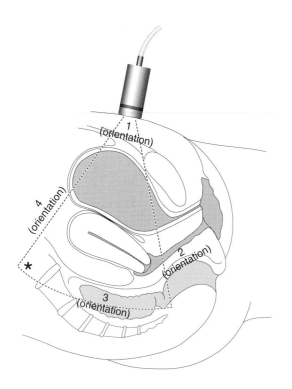

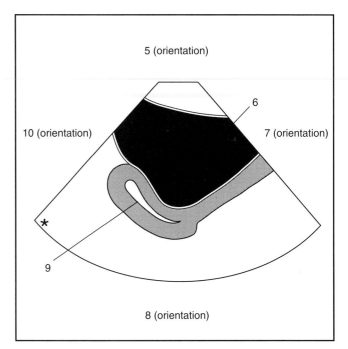

1 _____   6 _____

2 _____   7 _____

3 _____   8 _____

4 _____   9 _____

5 _____   10 _____

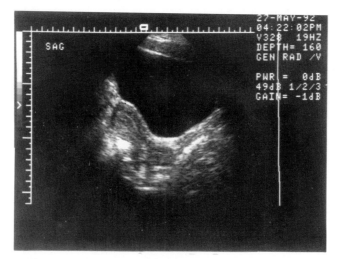

Figure 15–21. Transabdominal pelvic sagittal section.

DISPLAY MONITOR

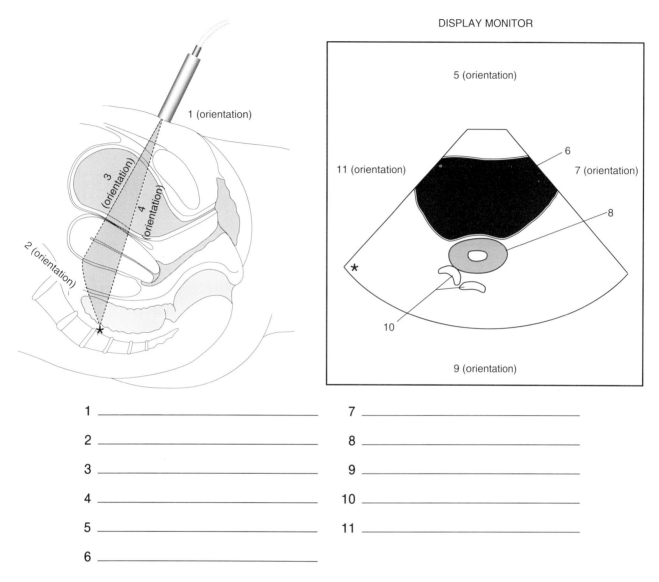

1 _____

2 _____

3 _____

4 _____

5 _____

6 _____

7 _____

8 _____

9 _____

10 _____

11 _____

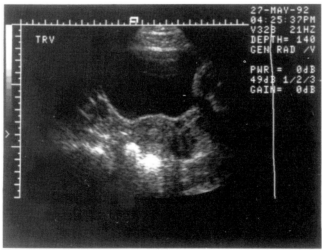

Figure 15–22. Transabdominal pelvic transverse section.

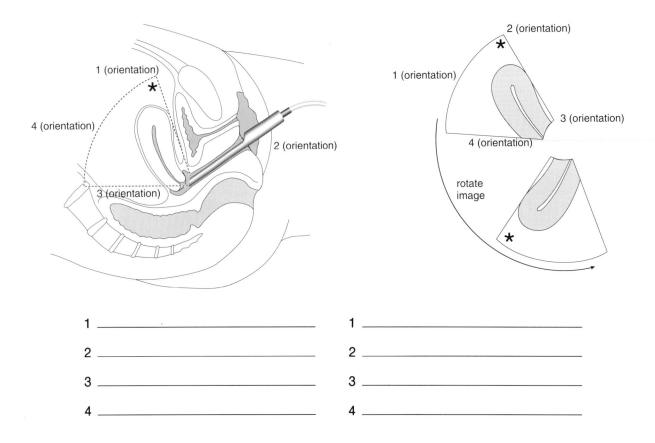

1 _____   1 _____

2 _____   2 _____

3 _____   3 _____

4 _____   4 _____

DISPLAY MONITOR

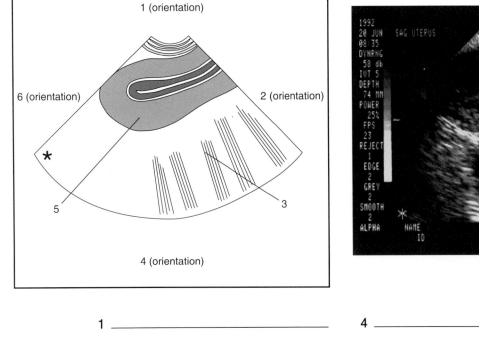

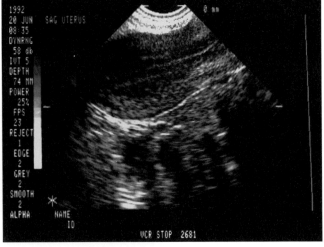

1 _____   4 _____

2 _____   5 _____

3 _____   6 _____

Figure 15–24. Transvaginal imaging in the coronal plane.

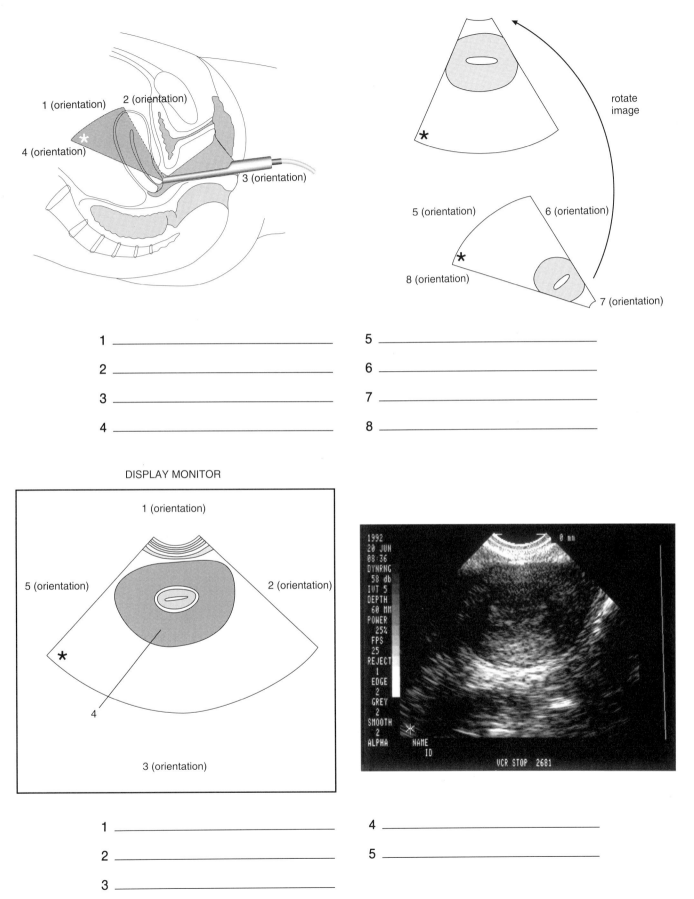

1 (orientation) 2 (orientation)
4 (orientation)
3 (orientation)

rotate image

5 (orientation) 6 (orientation)
8 (orientation)
7 (orientation)

1 _____ 5 _____

2 _____ 6 _____

3 _____ 7 _____

4 _____ 8 _____

DISPLAY MONITOR

1 (orientation)

5 (orientation)   2 (orientation)

4

3 (orientation)

1 _____ 4 _____

2 _____ 5 _____

3 _____

Figure 15–25. Transvaginal imaging in the coronal plane.

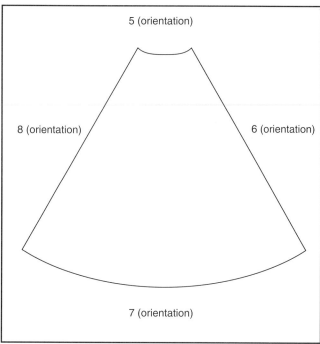

1 (orientation)

DISPLAY MONITOR

5 (orientation)

4 (orientation)

2 (orientation)

8 (orientation)

6 (orientation)

3 (orientation)

7 (orientation)

Figure 15–26. Transvaginal imaging: anterior approach.

1 _____   5 _____

2 _____   6 _____

3 _____   7 _____

4 _____   8 _____

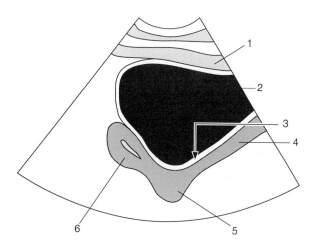

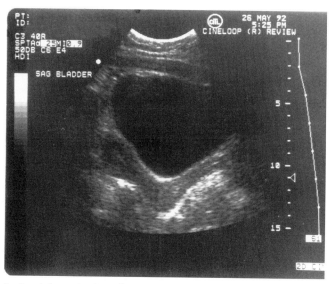

Figure 15–27. Transabdominal pelvic sagittal section.

1 _____   4 _____

2 _____   5 _____

3 _____   6 _____

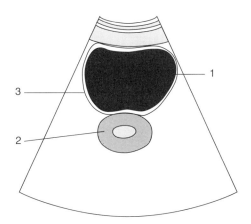
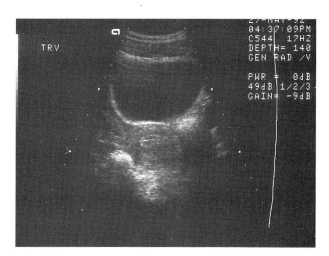

Figure 15-28. Transabdominal pelvic transverse section.

1 _____

2 _____

3 _____

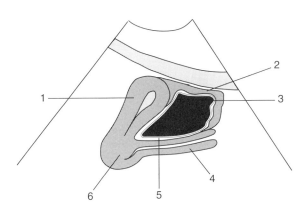
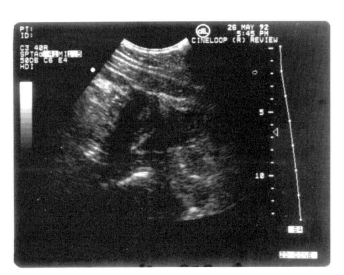

Figure 15-29. Transabdominal pelvic sagittal section.

1 _____   4 _____

2 _____   5 _____

3 _____   6 _____

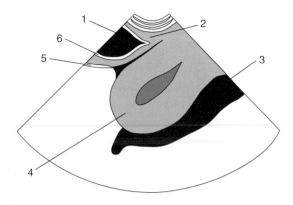
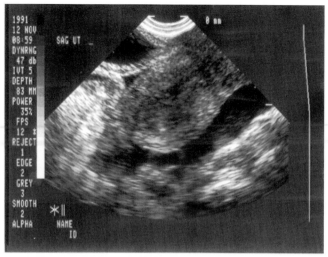

Figure 15–30.   Transvaginal sagittal section.

1 _____   4 _____

2 _____   5 _____

3 _____   6 _____

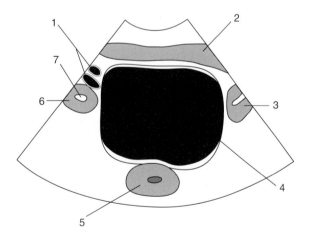
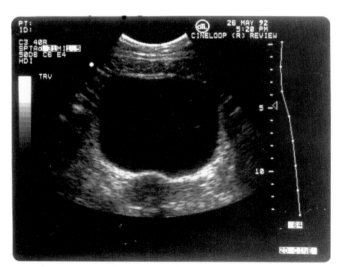

Figure 15–31.   Transabdominal pelvic transverse section.

1 _____   5 _____

2 _____   6 _____

3 _____   7 _____

4 _____

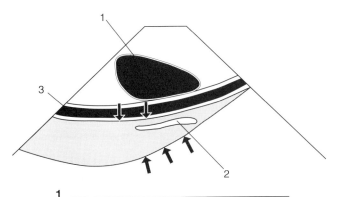

1 _____

2 _____

3 _____

4 Define the anatomic area indicated by the arrows _____

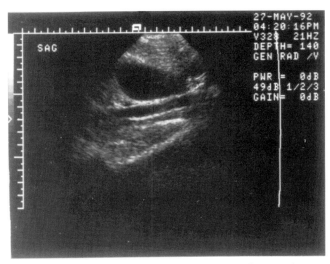

Figure 15-32. Transabdominal adnexa sagittal section.

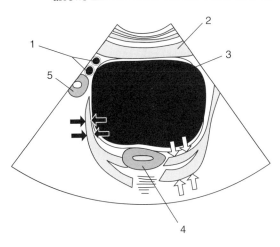

Figure 15-33. Transabdominal pelvic transverse section.

1 _____ 4 _____

2 _____ 5 _____

3 _____

6 Define the anatomic area indicated by the arrows _____

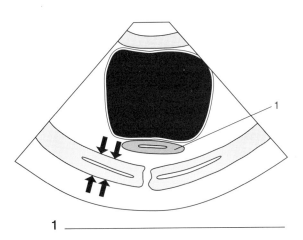

1 _____

2 Define the anatomic area indicated by the arrows _____

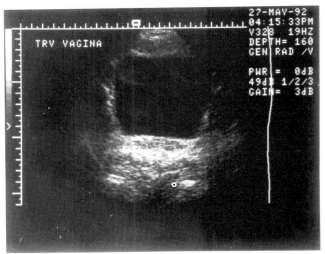

Figure 15-34. Transabdominal pelvic transverse section.

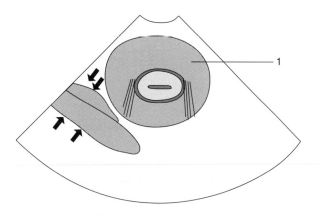

1 _____

2 Define the anatomic area indicated by the arrows _____

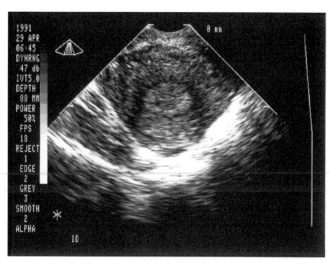

Figure 15-35. Transvaginal coronal section.

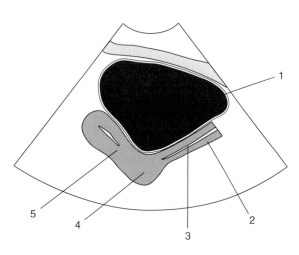

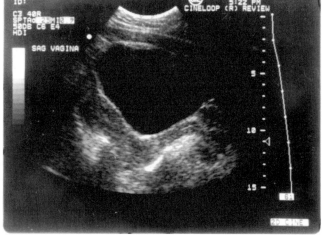

Figure 15-36. Transabdominal pelvic sagittal section.

1 _____ 4 _____

2 _____ 5 _____

3 _____

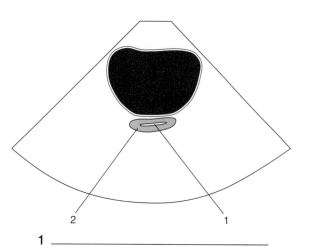

1 _____

2 _____

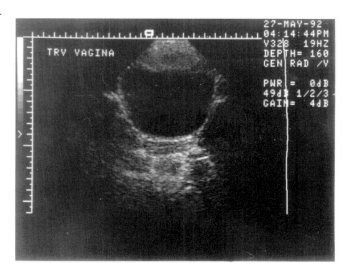

Figure 15-37. Transabdominal pelvic transverse section.

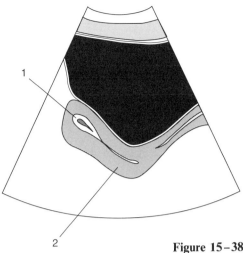

Figure 15-38. Transabdominal pelvic sagittal section.

1 _____

2 _____

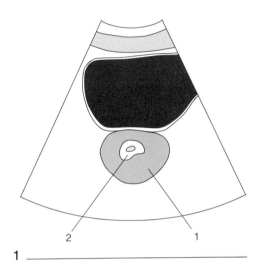

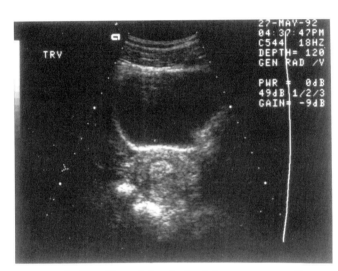

Figure 15-39. Transabdominal pelvic transverse section.

1 _____

2 _____

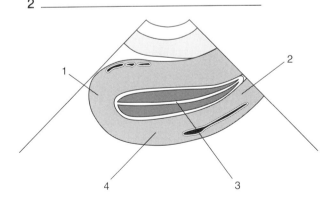

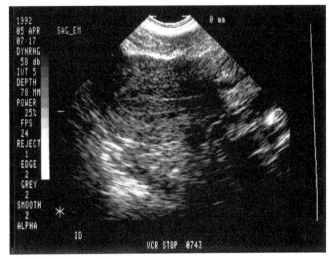

Figure 15-40. Transvaginal sagittal section.

1 _____   3 _____

2 _____   4 _____

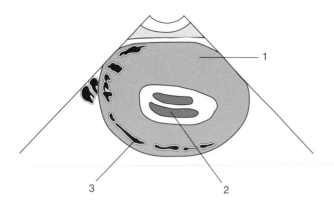
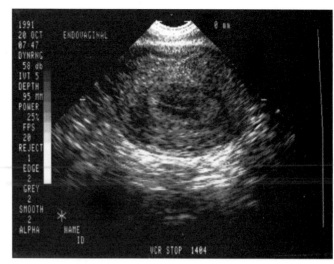

Figure 15–41. Transvaginal coronal section.

1 _____

2 _____

3 _____

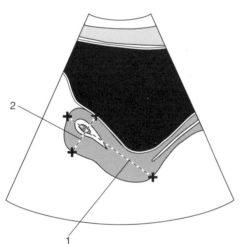
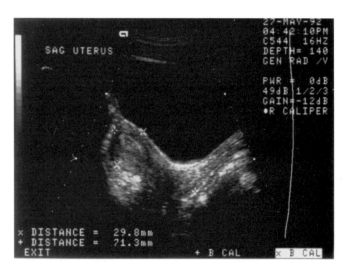

Figure 15–42. Uterine measurements sagittal section.

1 _____

2 _____

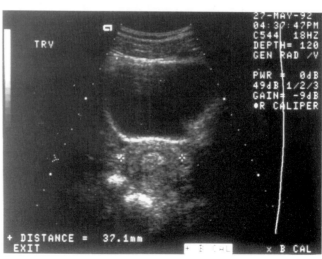

1 _____

Figure 15–43. Uterine measurement transverse section.

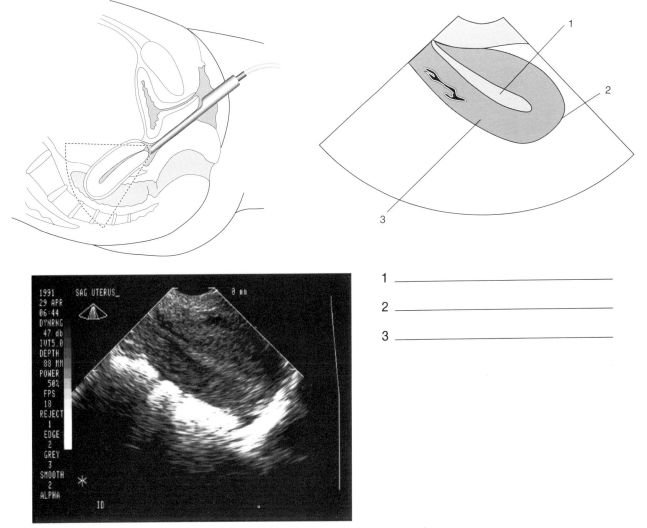

1	
2	
3	

Figure 15–44. Transvaginal sagittal section.

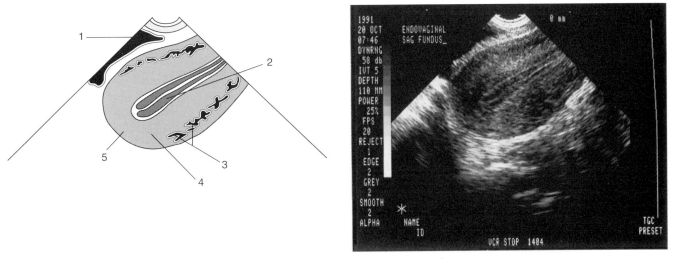

Figure 15–45. Transvaginal sagittal section.

1		4	
2		5	
3			

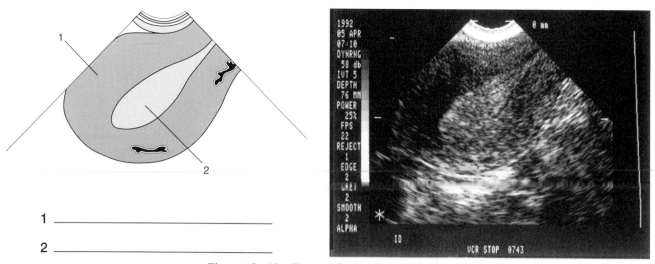

1 _____

2 _____

Figure 15–46. Transvaginal sagittal section.

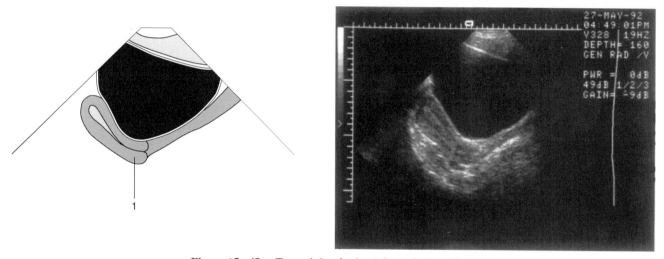

Figure 15–48. Transabdominal pelvic sagittal section.

1 _____

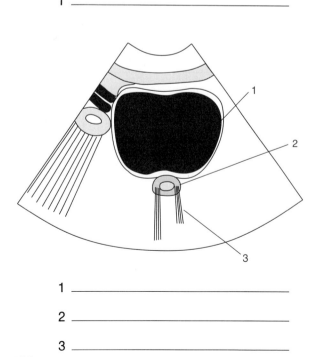

1 _____

2 _____

3 _____

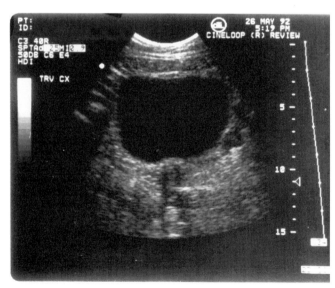

Figure 15–49. Transabdominal pelvic transverse section.

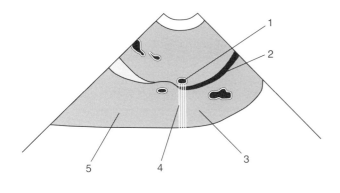
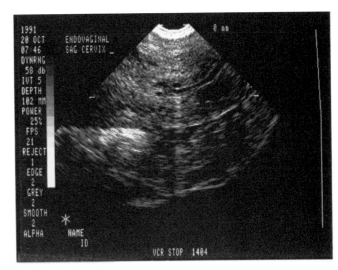

Figure 15–50. Transvaginal sagittal section.

1 _____   4 _____

2 _____   5 _____

3 _____

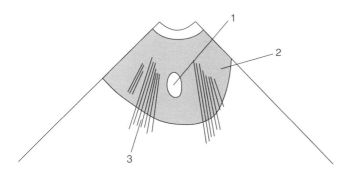
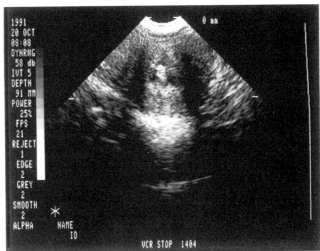

Figure 15–51. Transvaginal coronal section.

1 _____

2 _____

3 _____

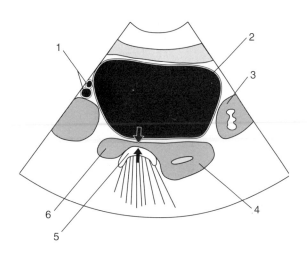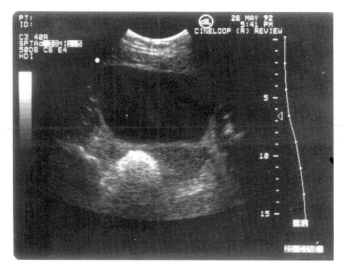

Figure 15–53. Transabdominal pelvic transverse section.

1 _____   4 _____

2 _____   5 _____

3 _____   6 _____

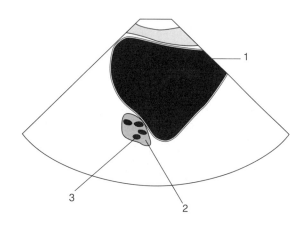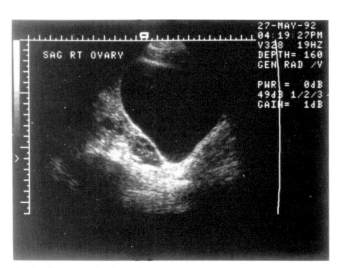

Figure 15–54. Transabdominal adnexa sagittal section.

1 _____

2 _____

3 _____

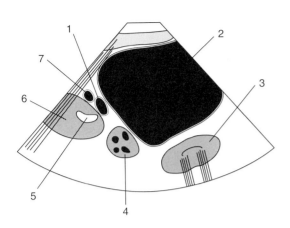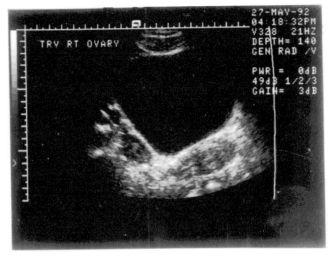

Figure 15–56. Transabdominal adnexa transverse section.

1 _____   5 _____

2 _____   6 _____

3 _____   7 _____

4 _____

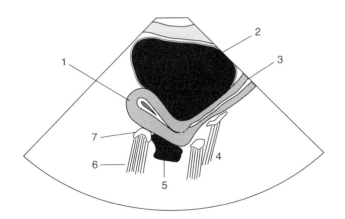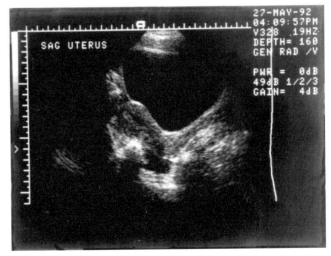

Figure 15–66. Transabdominal pelvic sagittal section.

1 _____   5 _____

2 _____   6 _____

3 _____   7 _____

4 _____

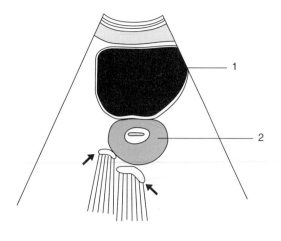
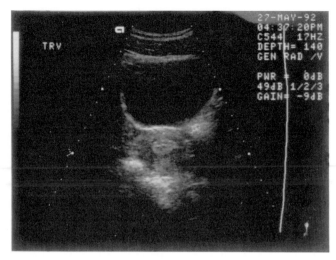

Figure 15-67. Transabdominal pelvic transverse section.

1 _____

2 _____

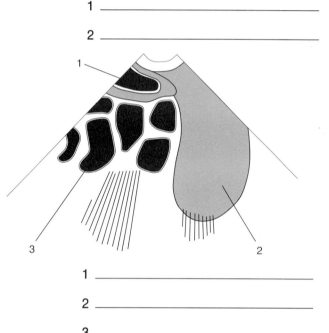

1 _____

2 _____

3 _____

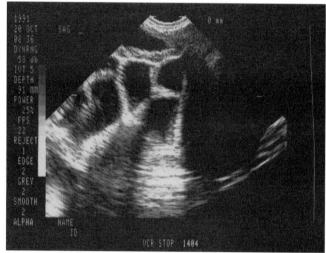

Figure 15-68. Transabdominal pelvic sagittal section.

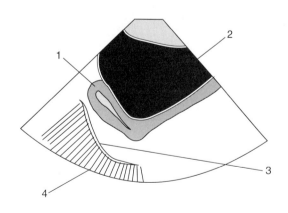

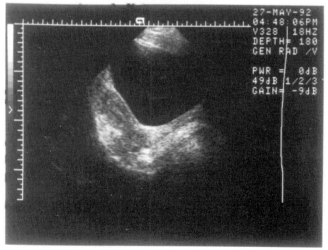

Figure 15-69. Transabdominal pelvic sagittal section.

1 _____   3 _____

2 _____   4 _____

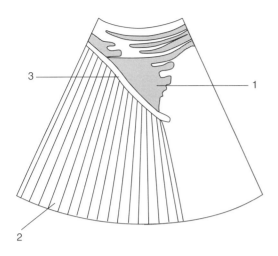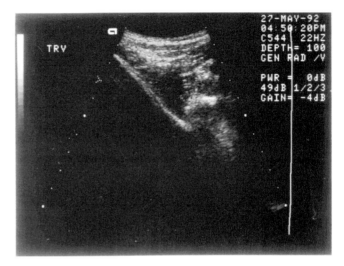

Figure 15–70. Transabdominal pelvic, transverse section.

1 _____

2 _____

3 _____

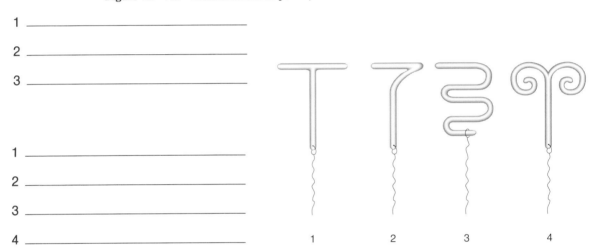

1 _____

2 _____

3 _____

4 _____

Figure 15–72. Intrauterine contraceptive devices.

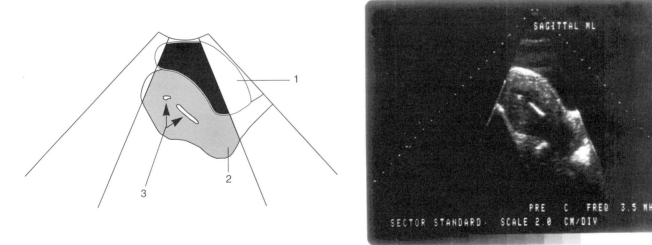

Figure 15–73. Transabdominal pelvic, IUD, sagittal section.

1 _____

2 _____

3 _____

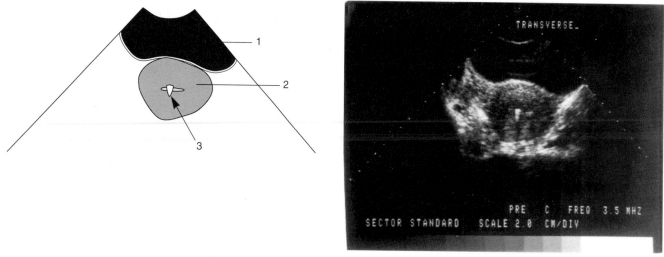

Figure 15–74. Transabdominal pelvic, IUD, transverse section.

1 _____

2 _____

3 _____

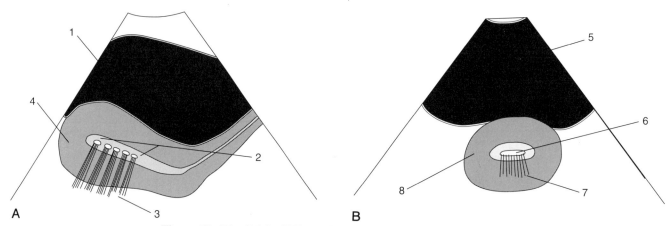

Figure 15–75. Pelvic, IUD, sagittal (A) and transverse (B) sections.

1 _____   5 _____

2 _____   6 _____

3 _____   7 _____

4 _____   8 _____

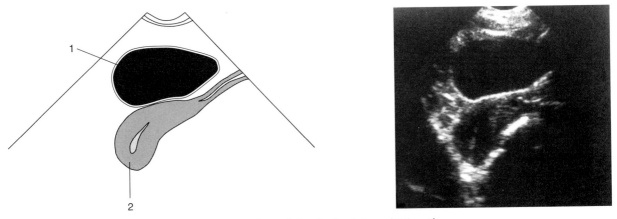

Figure 15-76. Transabdominal pelvic sagittal section.

1 _____

2 _____

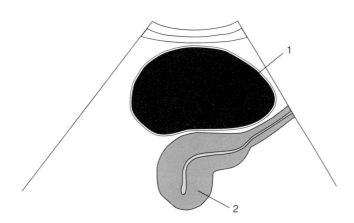

Figure 15-77. Transabdominal pelvic sagittal section.

1 _____

2 _____

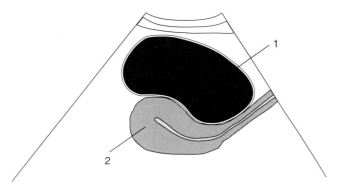

Figure 15-78. Transabdominal pelvic sagittal section.

1 _____

2 _____

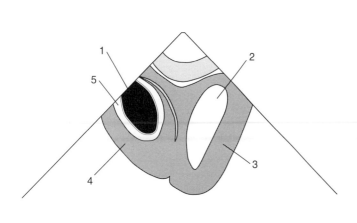
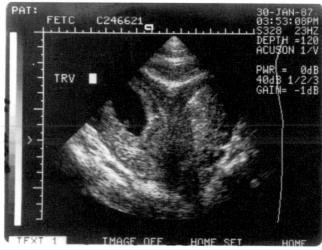

Figure 15–79. Transabdominal pelvic transverse section. Bicornate uterus.

1 _____   4 _____

2 _____   5 _____

3 _____

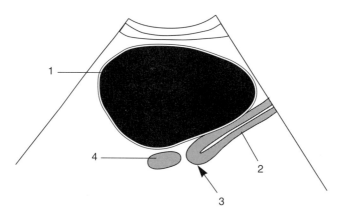

Figure 15–80. Transabdominal pelvic sagittal section. Post hysterectomy.

1 _____   3 _____

2 _____   4 _____

Chapter 16

FIRST TRIMESTER OBSTETRICS

REVIEW QUESTIONS

1. Progesterone is produced by the

a. uterus

b. pituitary gland

c. corpus luteum

d. none of the above

e. all of the above

2. Human chorionic gonadotropin is found in

a. urine

b. blood

c. amniotic fluid

d. a and b

e. b and c

3. Lacunae are structures within the

a. ovary

b. fetal brain

c. amnion

d. placenta

e. none of the above

4. The most accurate method of dating a gestation is the

a. sac size

b. crown rump length

c. biparietal diameter

d. femur length

e. yolk sac size

5. The yolk sac is

a. outside both chorion and amnion

b. inside both chorion and amnion

c. outside the amnion but inside the chorion

d. outside the chorion but inside the amnion

6. Fetal heart activity should usually be detected as early as the last menstrual period dating of

a. 3 weeks

b. 5 weeks

c. 7 weeks

d. 10 weeks

e. 12 weeks

7. Separation of chorion and amnion membranes at 14 weeks is

a. a sign of fetal death

b. a sign of twins

c. due to a large yolk sac

d. normal

e. none of the above

8. Which of the following is *not* a common indication for a first trimester ultrasound examination?

a. vaginal bleeding

b. size bigger than dates

c. size smaller than dates

d. pain

e. no sensation of fetal movement

9. The secondary yolk sac can

a. be bigger than the embryo

b. be cystic in appearance

c. be visualized before the embryo

d. disappear before the end of the first trimester

e. all of the above

10. A retroverted uterus

a. prevents pregnancy

b. is due to infection

c. may make the ultrasound examination more difficult

d. none of the above

e. is extremely rare

Identify the structures indicated in the following illustrations. These figures duplicate those found in **ULTRASONOGRAPHY: Introduction to Normal Structure and Functional Anatomy**. Refer to the textbook if you need help.

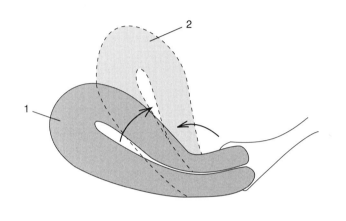
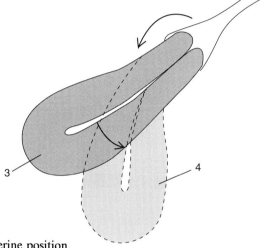

Figure 16–1. Variations in uterine position.

1 _____   3 _____

2 _____   4 _____

1 _____   5 _____

2 _____   6 _____

3 _____   7 _____

4 _____   8 _____

NORMAL EVENTS IN THE FIRST FOUR WEEKS OF GESTATION

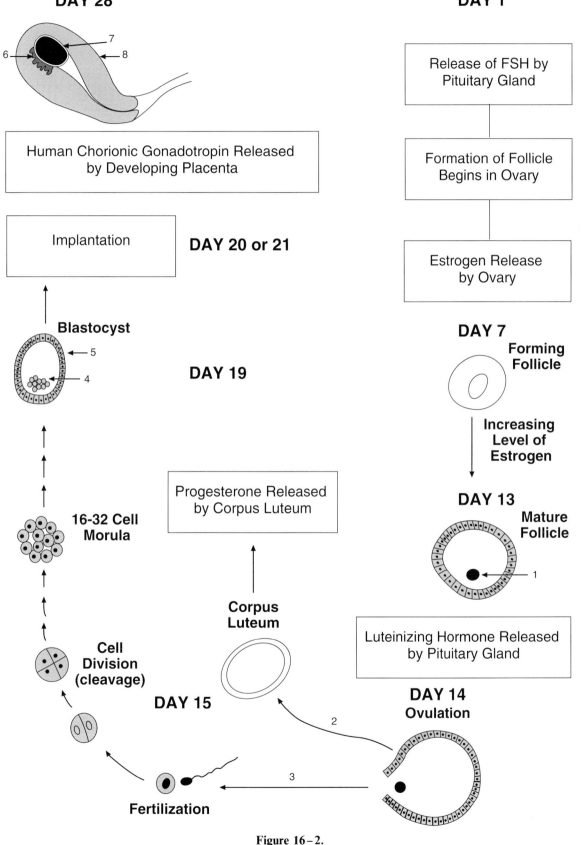

Figure 16–2.

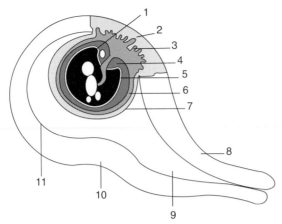

Figure 16–3. An 8 to 10 week gestational sac.

1 _____   7 _____

2 _____   8 _____

3 _____   9 _____

4 _____   10 _____

5 _____   11 _____

6 _____

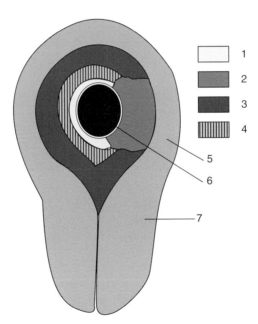

Figure 16–4. Decidual reaction.

1 _____   5 _____

2 _____   6 _____

3 _____   7 _____

4 _____

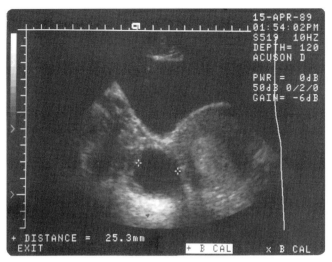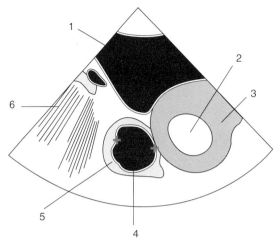

Figure 16–5. Pelvic transverse section.

1 _____ 4 _____

2 _____ 5 _____

3 _____ 6 _____

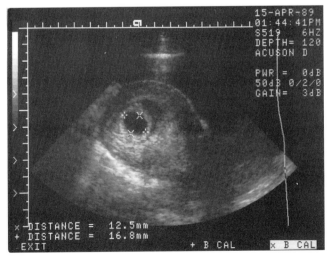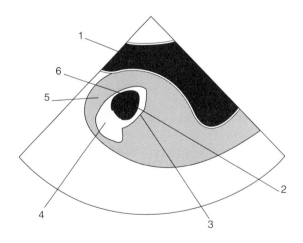

Figure 16–6. 5 week gestational sac longitudinal section.

1 _____ 4 _____

2 _____ 5 _____

3 _____ 6 _____

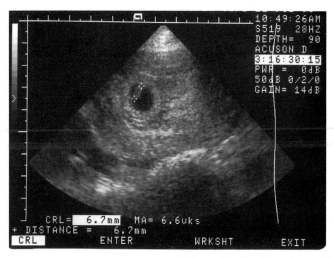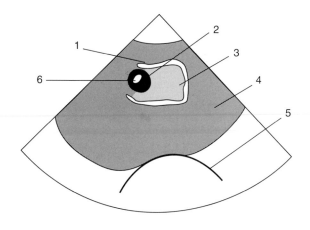

Figure 16-7. 5 week gestational sac transverse section.

1 _____   4 _____

2 _____   5 _____

3 _____   6 _____

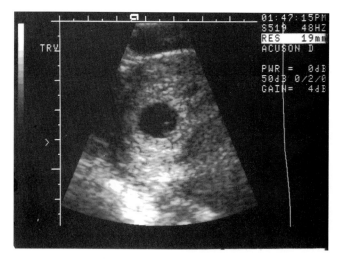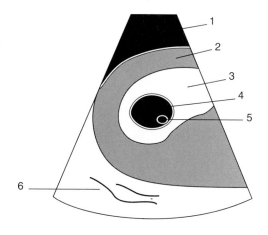

Figure 16-8. Secondary yolk sac at 6 weeks.

1 _____   4 _____

2 _____   5 _____

3 _____   6 _____

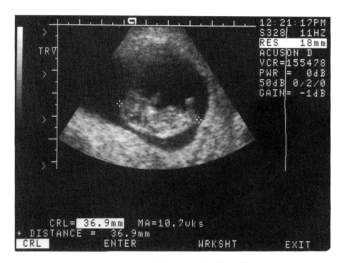 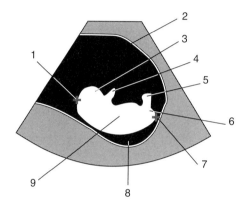

Figure 16–9. Crown-rump measurement in a 10.5 week embryo.

1 _____   6 _____

2 _____   7 _____

3 _____   8 _____

4 _____   9 _____

5 _____

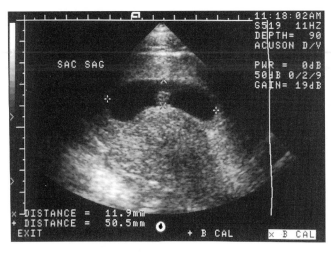
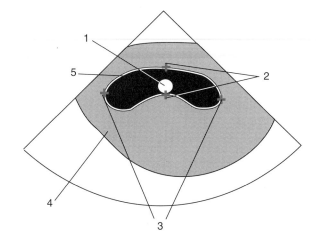

1 _____   4 _____

2 _____   5 _____

3 _____

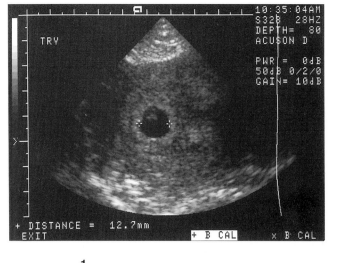
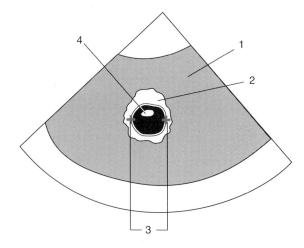

1 _____   3 _____

2 _____   4 _____

Figure 16–10. *Top,* Determination of sac size; longitudinal measurements; *bottom,* Determination of sac size: transverse measurement.

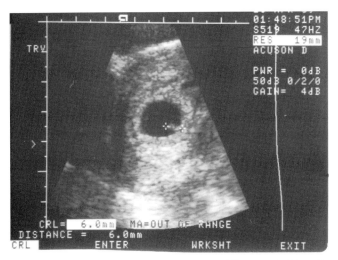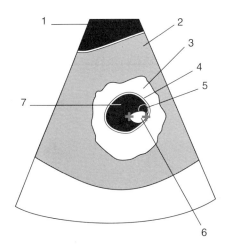

Figure 16-11. Gravid uterus.

1 _____   5 _____

2 _____   6 _____

3 _____   7 _____

4 _____

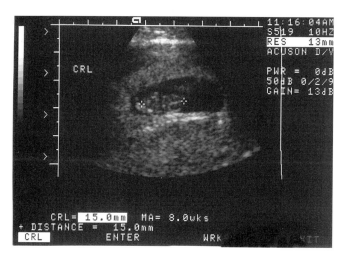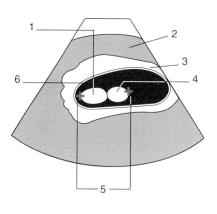

Figure 16-12. Gravid uterus.

1 _____   4 _____

2 _____   5 _____

3 _____   6 _____

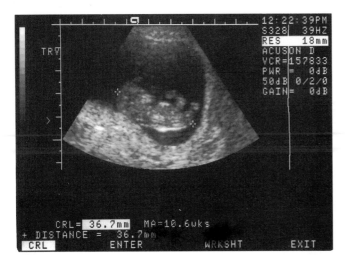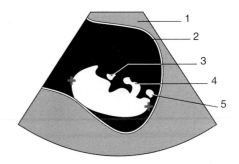

1 _____ 4 _____

2 _____ 5 _____

3 _____

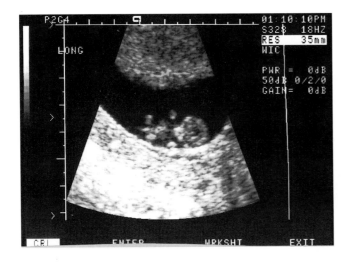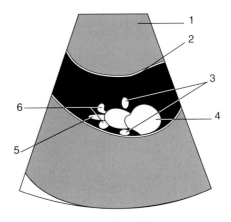

1 _____ 4 _____

2 _____ 5 _____

3 _____ 6 _____

Figure 16–13. *Top,* 10 to 11 week embryo; *bottom,* 9.5 week embryo.

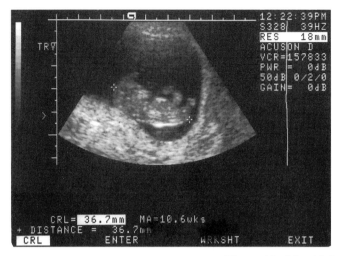
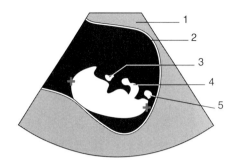

Figure 16–14. 10.5 week embryo.

1 _____   4 _____

2 _____   5 _____

3 _____   6 _____

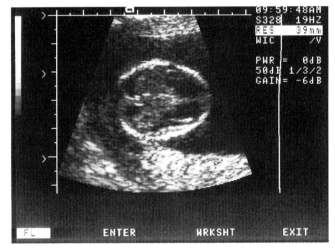
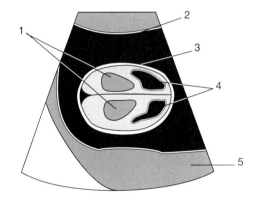

Figure 16–15. 12 week fetal skull.

1 _____   4 _____

2 _____   5 _____

3 _____

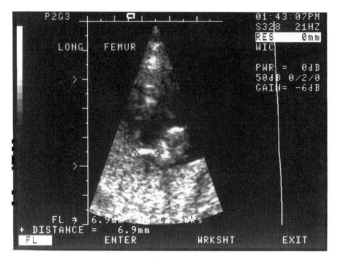 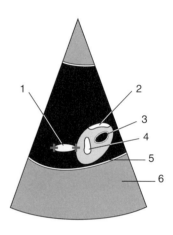

Figure 16–16. 12 week fetal femur.

1 _____ 4 _____

2 _____ 5 _____

3 _____ 6 _____

Chapter 17

SECOND AND THIRD TRIMESTER OBSTETRICS

REVIEW QUESTIONS

1. The fetal spine closes

a. from head to rump

b. uniformly, all at once

c. from ends to middle

d. from middle to ends

e. from rump to head

2. Cerebrospinal fluid is produced in the fetus by the

a. cerebellum

b. pons

c. choroid plexus

d. spine and brain

e. meninges

3. The fetal lungs can function as early as

a. 15 weeks

b. 20 weeks

c. 25 weeks

d. 35 weeks

e. none of the above

4. The umbilical cord has

a. one vessel

b. two vessels

c. three vessels

d. four vessels

e. six vessels

5. A grade III placenta may have

a. cystic areas

b. calcification

c. segments

d. calcified base plate

e. all of the above

6. A grade I placenta may have

a. cystic areas

b. calcification

c. segments

d. calcified base plate

e. none of the above

Identify the structures indicated in the following illustrations. These figures duplicate those found in **ULTRASONOGRAPHY: Introduction to Normal Structure and Functional Anatomy**. Refer to the textbook if you need help.

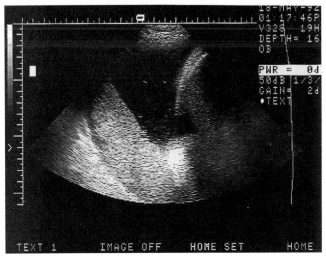
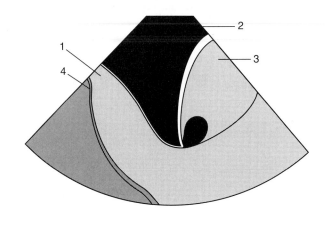

Figure 17-1. 18 week gestation.

1 _____   3 _____

2 _____   4 _____

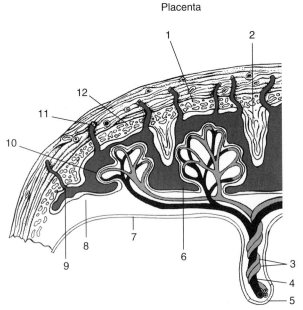

Figure 17-2. Maternal-fetal circulatory pattern in the placenta.

1 _____

2 _____

3 _____

4 _____

5 _____

6 _____

7 _____

8 _____

9 _____

10 _____

11 _____

12 _____

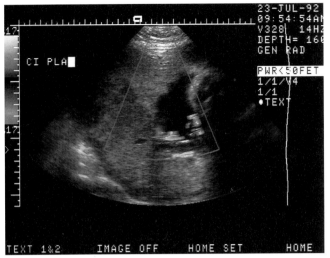 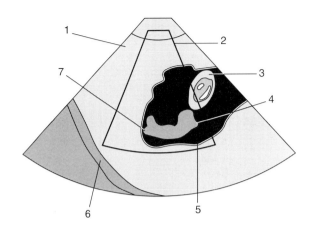

Figure 17–3. Color flow demonstration of placental cord insertion site.

1 _____   5 _____

2 _____   6 _____

3 _____   7 _____

4 _____

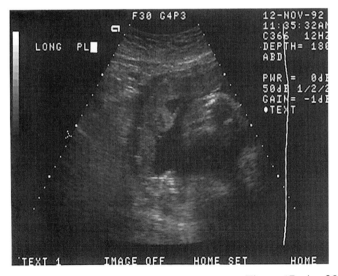 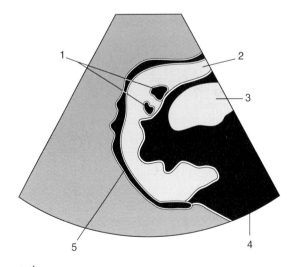

Figure 17–4. 25 week gestation.

1 _____   4 _____

2 _____   5 _____

3 _____

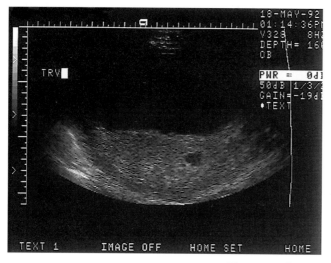
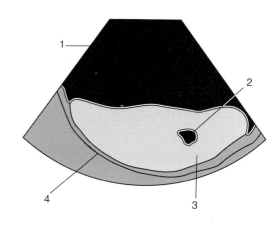

Figure 17–5. 32 week gestation.

1 _____   3 _____

2 _____   4 _____

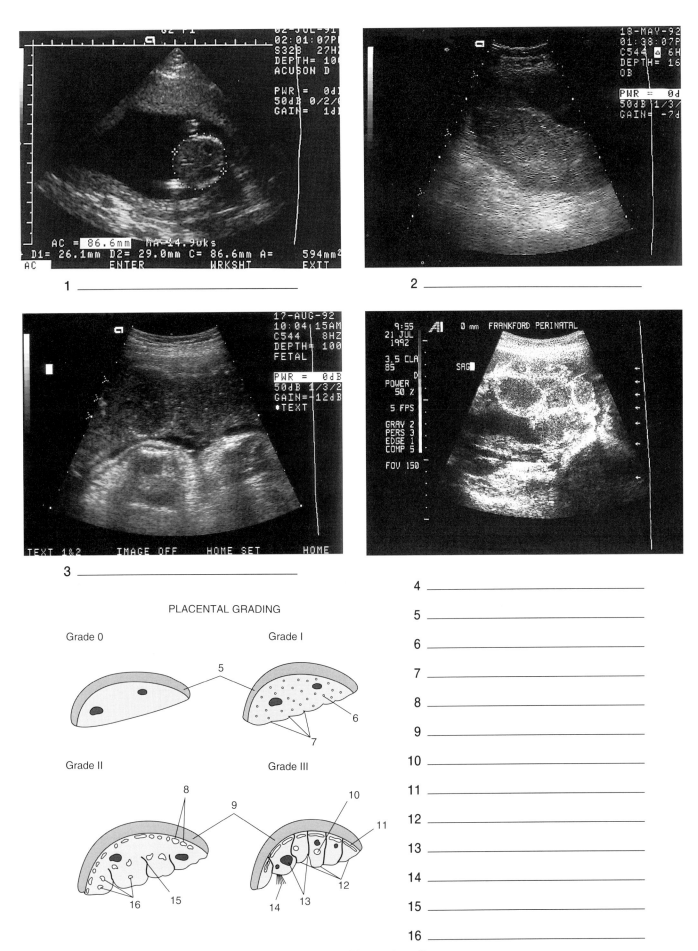

1 _____

2 _____

3 _____

4 _____

5 _____

6 _____

7 _____

8 _____

9 _____

10 _____

11 _____

12 _____

13 _____

14 _____

15 _____

16 _____

PLACENTAL GRADING

Grade 0   Grade I

Grade II   Grade III

Figure 17-6. Placental grading.

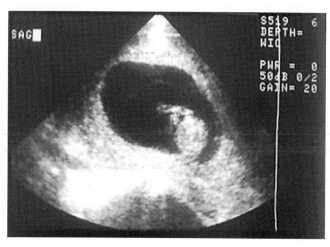 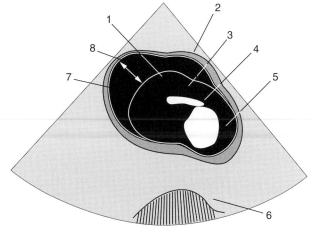

Figure 17–7. 14 week gestation.

1 _____   5 _____

2 _____   6 _____

3 _____   7 _____

4 _____   8 _____

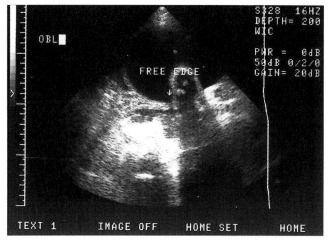 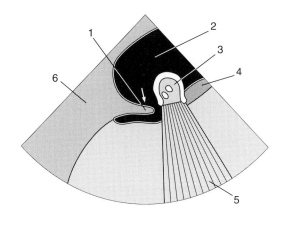

Figure 17–8. 30 week gestation.

1 _____   4 _____

2 _____   5 _____

3 _____   6 _____

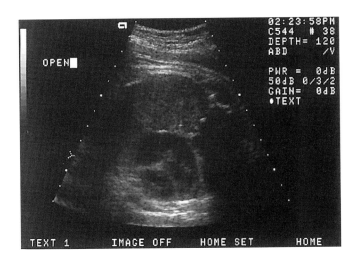

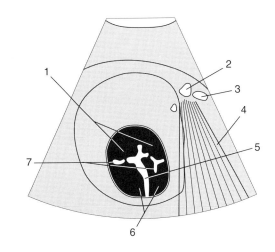

1 _____   5 _____

2 _____   6 _____

3 _____   7 _____

4 _____

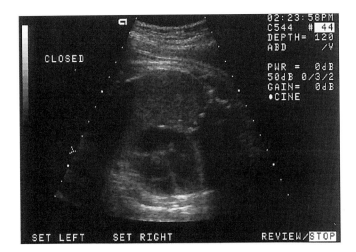

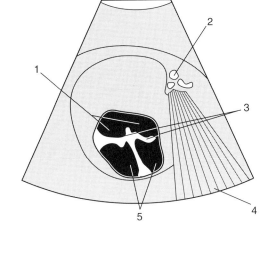

1 _____   4 _____

2 _____   5 _____

3 _____

Figure 17–9. 33 week fetal heart.

Figure continues on the following page

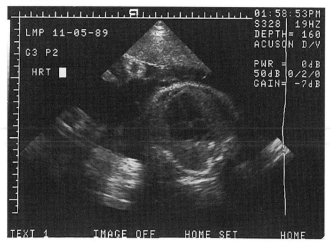

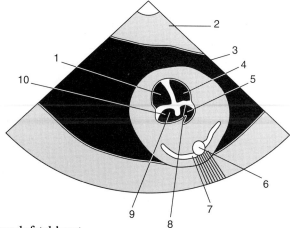

Figure 17–9. *Continued.* 34 week fetal heart.

1 _____	6 _____
2 _____	7 _____
3 _____	8 _____
4 _____	9 _____
5 _____	10 _____

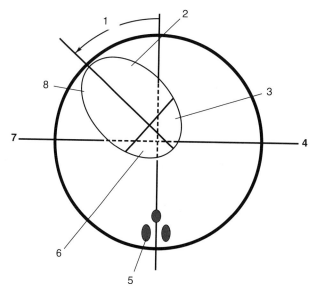

Figure 17–10. Position of the fetal heart.

1 _____	5 _____
2 _____	6 _____
3 _____	7 _____
4 _____	8 _____

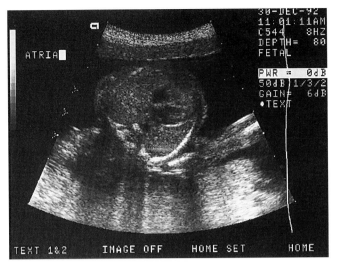 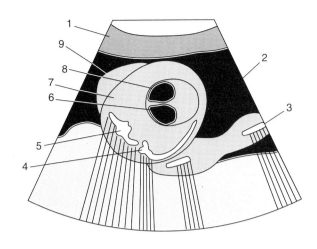

27 week gestation.

1 _____ 6 _____

2 _____ 7 _____

3 _____ 8 _____

4 _____ 9 _____

5 _____

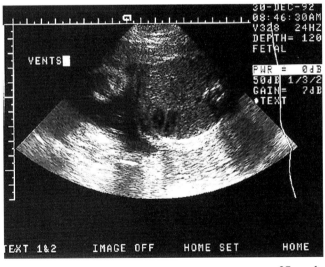 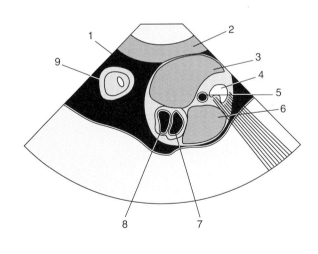

27 week gestation.

1 _____ 6 _____

2 _____ 7 _____

3 _____ 8 _____

4 _____ 9 _____

5 _____

Figure 17–11.

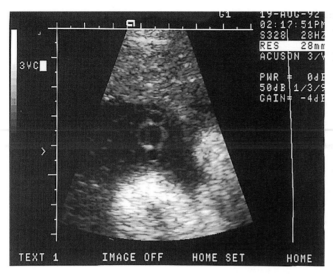 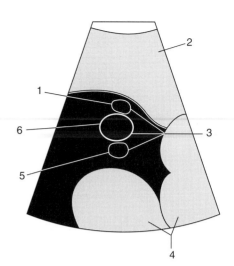

Figure 17-12. Umbilical cord.

1 _____   4 _____

2 _____   5 _____

3 _____   6 _____

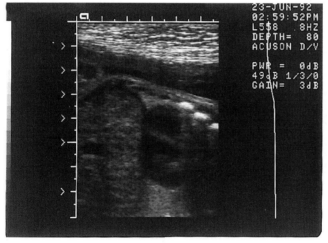 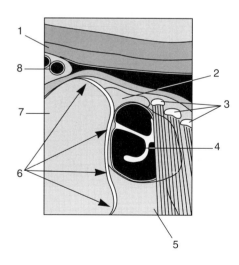

Figure 17-13. 27 week gestation.

1 _____   5 _____

2 _____   6 _____

3 _____   7 _____

4 _____   8 _____

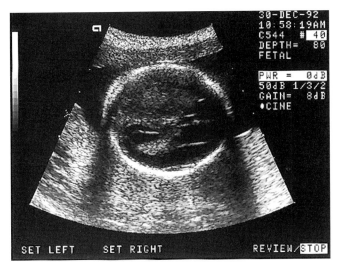 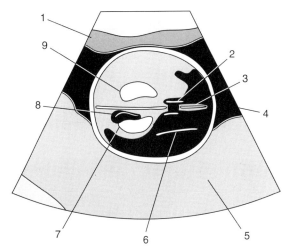

Figure 17–14. 18 week gestation/fetal head.

1 _____   6 _____

2 _____   7 _____

3 _____   8 _____

4 _____   9 _____

5 _____

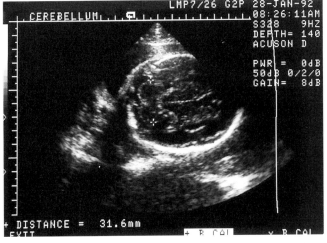 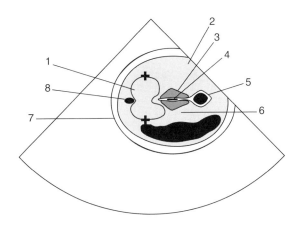

Figure 17–15. 19 week gestation/fetal head.

1 _____   5 _____

2 _____   6 _____

3 _____   7 _____

4 _____   8 _____

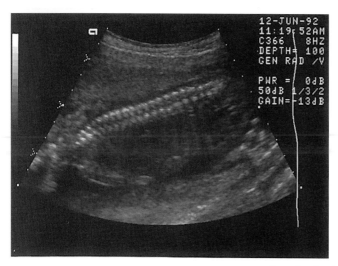
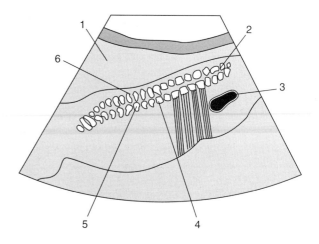

Longitudinal fetal spine.

1 _____   4 _____

2 _____   5 _____

3 _____   6 _____

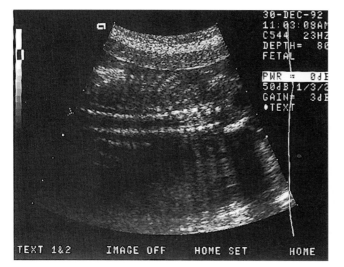
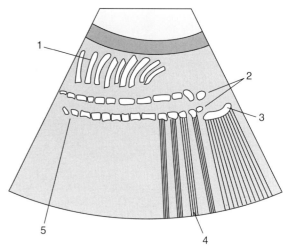

Coronal view fetal spine.

1 _____   4 _____

2 _____   5 _____

3 _____

Figure 17–16.

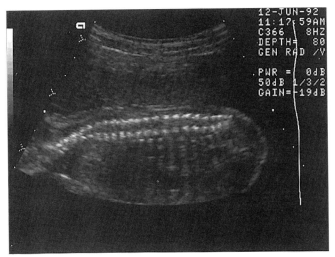
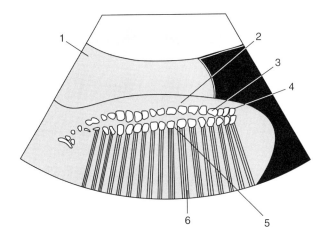

Longitudinal fetal spine.

1 _____   4 _____

2 _____   5 _____

3 _____   6 _____

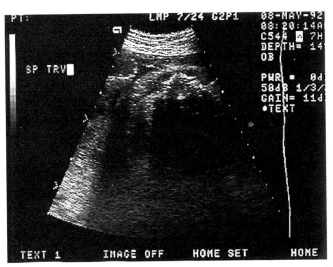
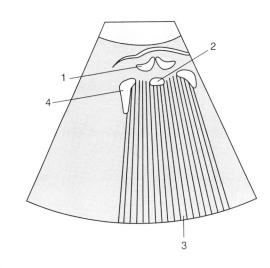

Transverse fetal spine.

1 _____   3 _____

2 _____   4 _____

Figure 17–17.

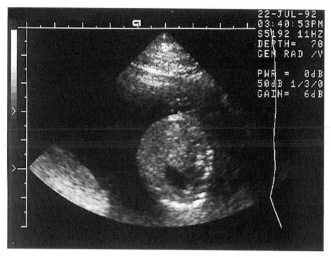 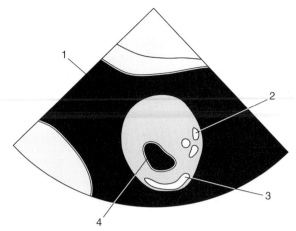

35 week gestation transverse section.

1 _____   3 _____

2 _____   4 _____

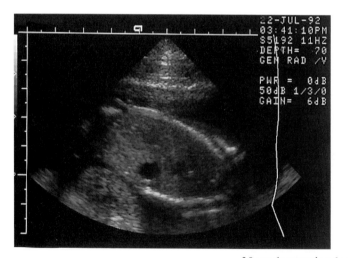 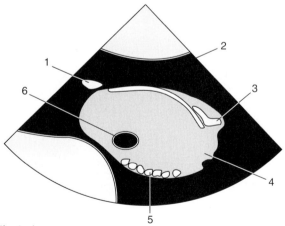

35 week gestation longitudinal view.

1 _____   4 _____

2 _____   5 _____

3 _____   6 _____

Figure 17–18.

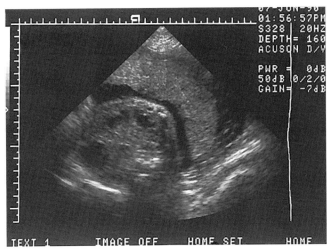
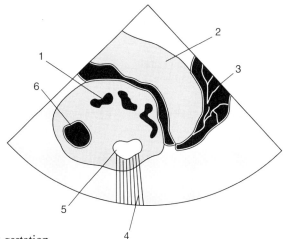

Figure 17–19. 30 week gestation.

1 _____   4 _____

2 _____   5 _____

3 _____   6 _____

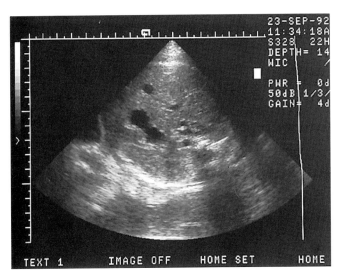
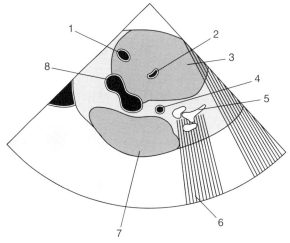

Figure 17–20. 27 week gestation.

1 _____   5 _____

2 _____   6 _____

3 _____   7 _____

4 _____   8 _____

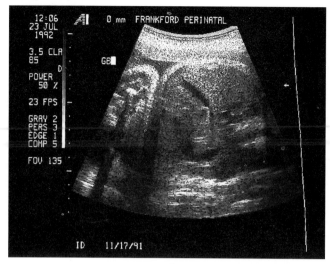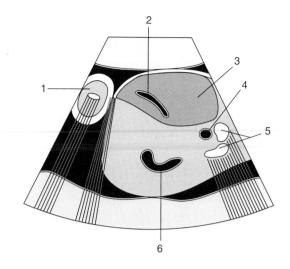

Figure 17–21. Fetal abdomen.

1 _____   4 _____

2 _____   5 _____

3 _____   6 _____

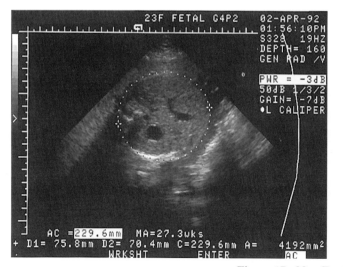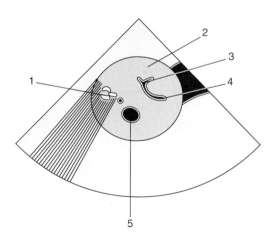

Figure 17–22. Fetal abdomen.

1 _____   4 _____

2 _____   5 _____

3 _____

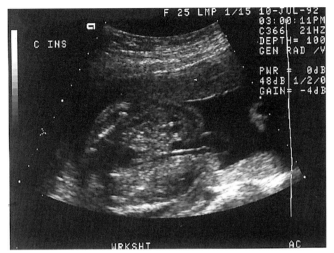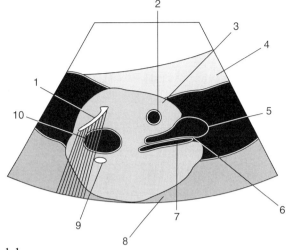

Figure 17–23. Fetal abdomen.

1 _____	6 _____
2 _____	7 _____
3 _____	8 _____
4 _____	9 _____
5 _____	10 _____

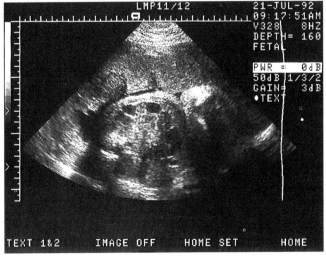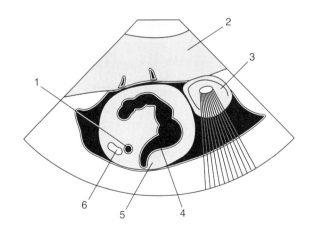

Figure 17–24. Fetal abdomen.

1 _____	4 _____
2 _____	5 _____
3 _____	6 _____

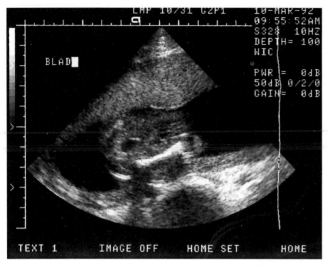
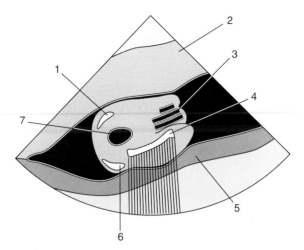

Figure 17-25. Fetal pelvis.

1 _____   5 _____

2 _____   6 _____

3 _____   7 _____

4 _____

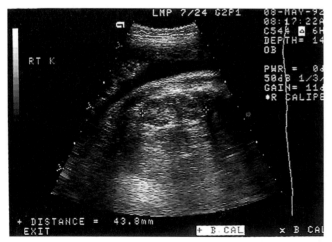
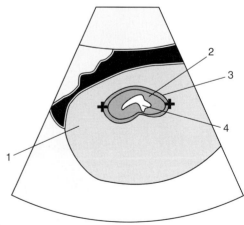

Fetal kidney longitudinal view.

1 _____   3 _____

2 _____   4 _____

Figure 17-26.

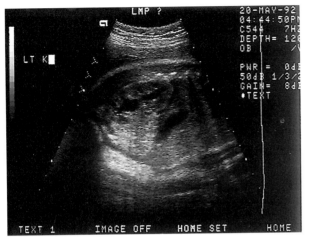 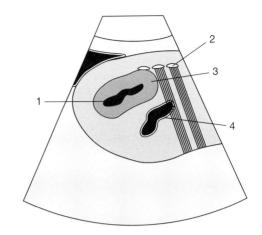

Fetal kidney.

1 _____   3 _____

2 _____   4 _____

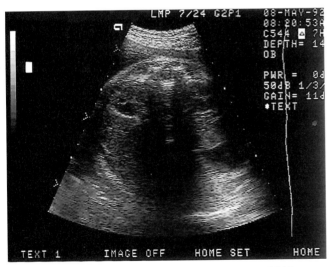 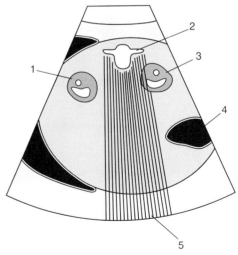

Fetal kidneys transverse view.

1 _____   4 _____

2 _____   5 _____

3 _____

Figure 17–26. *Continued*

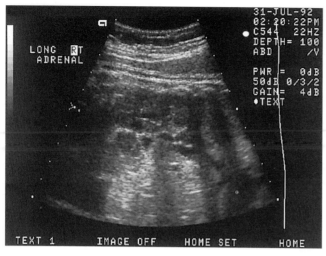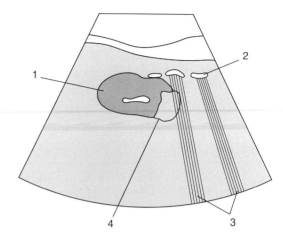

Fetal adrenal gland longitudinal view.

1 _____   3 _____

2 _____   4 _____

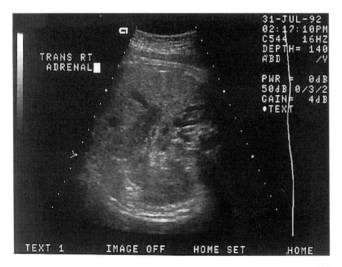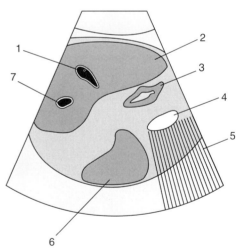

Fetal adrenal gland transverse view.

1 _____   5 _____

2 _____   6 _____

3 _____   7 _____

4 _____

Figure 17–27.

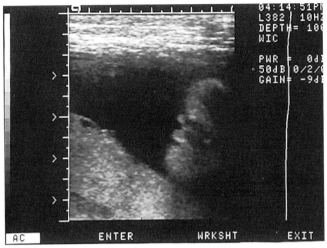 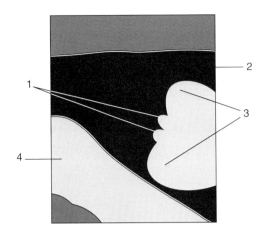

32 week gestation/female genitalia.

1 _____   3 _____

2 _____   4 _____

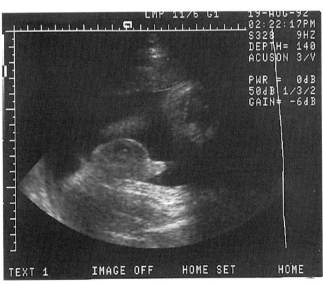 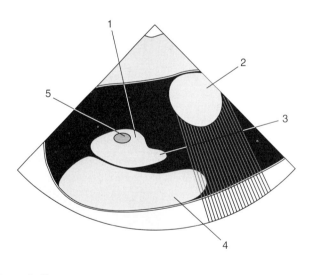

30 week gestation/male genitalia.

1 _____   4 _____

2 _____   5 _____

3 _____

Figure 17–28.

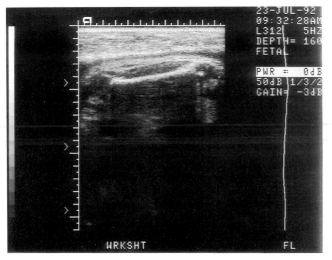
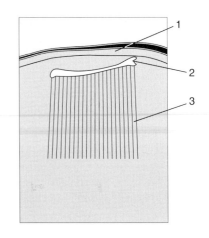

Fetal femur.

1 _____

2 _____

3 _____

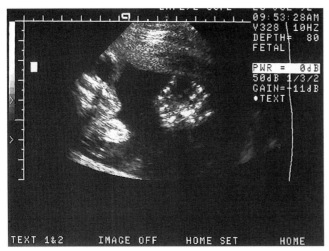
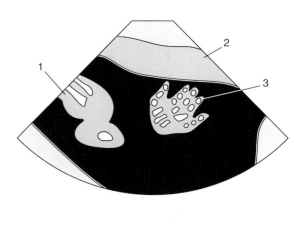

33 week gestation/fetal hand.

1 _____

2 _____

3 _____

Figure 17–29.

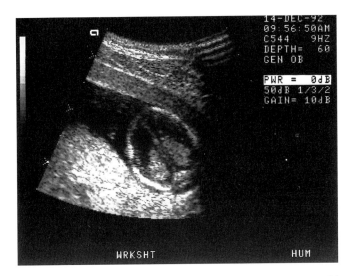 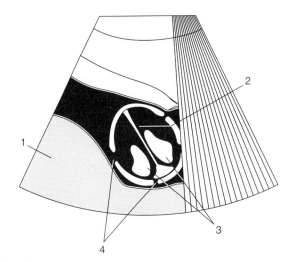

Figure 17–30. Fetal head.

1 _____   3 _____

2 _____   4 _____

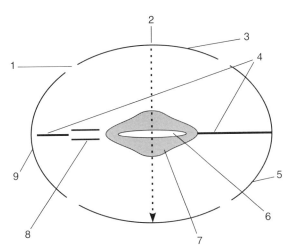

Figure 17–31. Biparietal diameter measurement.

1 _____   6 _____

2 _____   7 _____

3 _____   8 _____

4 _____   9 _____

5 _____

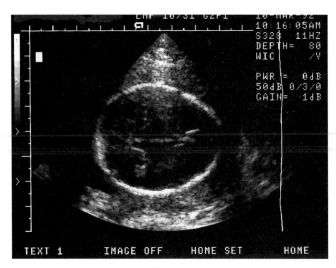

BPD image.

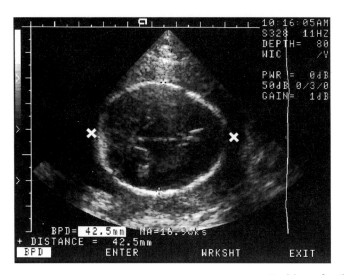

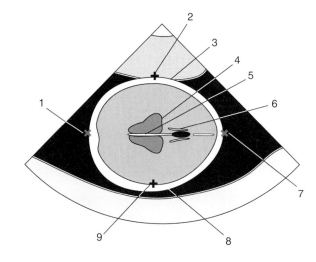

Position of calipers for OFD.

1 _____   6 _____

2 _____   7 _____

3 _____   8 _____

4 _____   9 _____

5 _____

Figure 17–32.

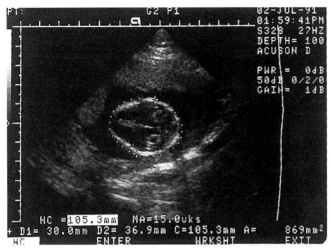 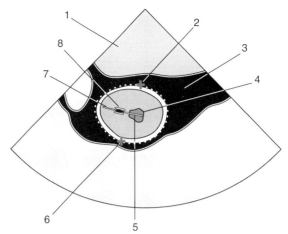

Position of calipers for BPD.

1 _____   5 _____

2 _____   6 _____

3 _____   7 _____

4 _____   8 _____

Figure 17–32. *Continued*

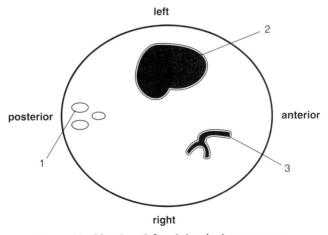

Figure 17–33. Level for abdominal measurement.

1 _____

2 _____

3 _____

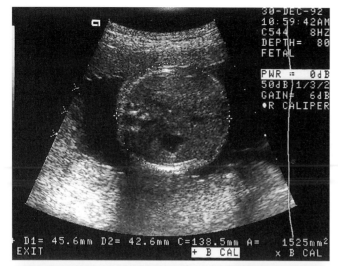

Fetal abdomen image for circumference measurement.

D1= 45.6mm D2= 42.6mm C=138.5mm A=   1525mm²

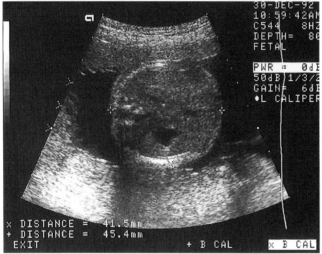

Position of calipers for average abdominal diameter measurements.

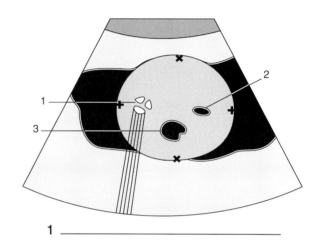

1 _____

2 _____

3 _____

Figure 17–34.

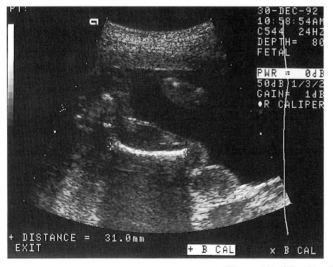

Figure 17–35. Fetal femur measurement.

1 _____   5 _____

2 _____   6 _____

3 _____   7 _____

4 _____

Chapter 18

OBSTETRIC SONOGRAPHY/SPECIAL SITUATIONS

REVIEW QUESTIONS

1. The maximum score on the ultrasound portion of a biophysical profile is

a. 4 points

b. 6 points

c. 8 points

d. 10 points

e. 25 points

2. Fetal respiration on a biophysical profile must take place for

a. 1 minute

b. 10 minutes

c. 15 minutes

d. 30 minutes

e. Fetal respiration is not part of the biophysical profile

3. The lecithin-sphingomyelin (L-S) ratio is used to

a. determine whether abnormalities are present

b. rule out infections

c. determine cardiac activity

d. determine lung maturity

e. date the early pregnancy for chorionic villus sampling (CVS)

4. Which of the following procedures is done earliest in a pregnancy?

a. CVS

b. amniocentesis for L-S ratio

c. amniocentesis for genetic analysis

d. cord Doppler

e. cord transfusions

5. Amniocentesis is associated with which of the following risks?

a. infection

b. needle injury

c. premature delivery

d. a and b

e. a, b, and c

Identify the structures indicated in the following illustrations. These figures duplicate those found in **ULTRASONOGRAPHY: Introduction to Normal Structure and Functional Anatomy**. Refer to the textbook if you need help.

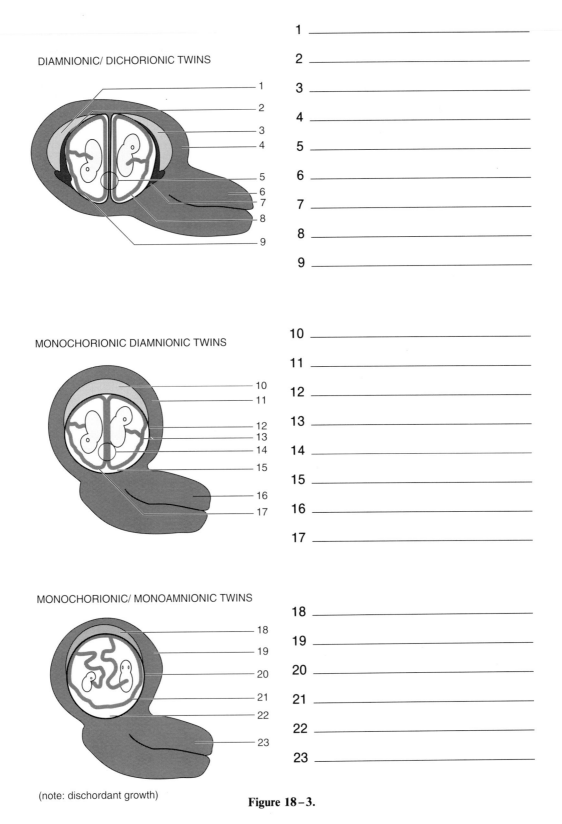

DIAMNIONIC/ DICHORIONIC TWINS

MONOCHORIONIC DIAMNIONIC TWINS

MONOCHORIONIC/ MONOAMNIONIC TWINS

(note: dischordant growth)

1 _____

2 _____

3 _____

4 _____

5 _____

6 _____

7 _____

8 _____

9 _____

10 _____

11 _____

12 _____

13 _____

14 _____

15 _____

16 _____

17 _____

18 _____

19 _____

20 _____

21 _____

22 _____

23 _____

Figure 18–3.

Chapter 19

THE THYROID AND PARATHYROID GLANDS

REVIEW QUESTIONS

1. The thyroid is an endocrine gland that secretes three hormones, which are

    a. triiodothyronine (T4), thyroxine (T5), and calcitonin

    b. triiodothyronine (T3), thyroxine (T4), and calcitonin

    c. triiodothyronine (T3), thyroxine (T4), and iron

    d. triiodothyronine (T3), thyroxine (T7), and iron

2. Each of the following statements regarding the thyroid gland is true *except*

    a. it lies anterior to the trachea

    b. it is composed of right and left lobes

    c. a pyramidal lobe is present in approximately 15 to 30% of the population

    d. it is an exocrine gland

3. The average weight of the thyroid gland is approximately

    a. 2–15 grams

    b. 30–40 grams

    c. 25–35 grams

    d. 10–15 grams

4. Which one of the following statements is *not* true regarding the thyroid gland

    a. measures approximately 4–6 cm in length, 2.0 to 3.0 cm in anteroposterior diameter, and 1.5 to 2 cm in width

    b. in cross-section is outlined laterally by the common carotid artery and the internal jugular vein

    c. the isthmus measures approximately 1-2 mm in anteroposterior diameter

    d. plays a major role in growth and development, and regulates basal metabolism by the synthesis, storage, and secretion of thyroid hormones

5. Neck muscles located anterolateral to the thyroid gland include all of the following *except*

    a. the sternothyroid and sternohyoid

    b. the longus colli

    c. the sternocleidomastoid

    d. the omohyoid and thyrohyoid

6. The sonographic appearance of the normal thyroid gland is uniformly

    a. hypoechoic with scattered hyperechoic regions

    b. echogenic with medium level echoes similar to the liver and testes

    c. hyperechoic with high level echoes

    d. hypoechoic with medium level echoes

7. The following statements are true regarding the sonographic appearance of neck muscles and the esophagus *except*

    a. the esophagus appears hypoechoic with an echogenic center representing mucosa

    b. the longus colli muscle is hyperechoic compared with the thyroid gland

    c. the sternocleidomastoid muscle is hypoechoic compared with the thyroid gland

    d. the infrahyoid muscles are hypoechoic relative to the thyroid gland

8. The secretion of triiodothyronine (T3), thyroxine (T4), and calcitonin is regulated by the

a. liver and pituitary gland

b. hypothalamus and the pituitary gland

c. hypothalamus only

d. parafollicular cells (C cells)

9. The thyroid gland is composed of follicles filled with a substance called

a. thyrotropin

b. colloid

c. calcitonin

d. none of the above

10. Each of the following statements regarding parathyroid glands is true *except*

a. most people (about 80 to 85%) have four parathyroid glands located in a symmetric position (two upper and two lower)

b. parathyroid glands are situated posterior to the thyroid gland

c. parathyroid glands may be intrathyroidal

d. ectopic parathyroid glands represent approximately 5% of the total

11. Parathyroid glands develop from the

a. first and second pharyngeal pouches

b. third and fifth pharyngeal pouches

c. third and fourth pharyngeal pouches

d. none of the above

12. Which of the following statements is *not* true regarding parathyroid glands?

a. ectopic parathyroid glands represent approximately 15 to 20% of the total

b. ectopic locations include the carotid bulb, retroesophageal, thymus, and intrathyroidal

c. normal parathyroid glands measure approximately 5 to 7 mm in length, 3 to 4 mm in width, and 1 to 2 mm in thickness

d. the shape of parathyroid glands varies; they are generally elongated

13. The sonographic appearance of parathyroid glands is

a. always hyperechoic compared to the thyroid gland

b. hypoechoic to anechoic without through transmission

c. anechoic with through transmission

d. none of the above

14. Each of the following statements regarding parathyroid glands is true *except*

a. normal parathyroid glands are usually not seen by sonography

b. parathyroid glands are situated posterior to the thyroid gland and anterior to the longus colli muscle

c. a prominent longus colli muscle may be mistaken for a parathyroid adenoma

d. the minor neurovascular bundle is never mistaken for a parathyroid adenoma

15. Each of the following statements regarding parathyroid gland physiology is true *except*

a. parathyroid glands secrete parathyroid hormone, also called PTH or parathormone

b. parathyroid glands maintain homeostastis of blood calcium by promoting calcium absorption into the blood and preventing hypocalcemia

c. when serum calcium levels are low, the parathyroid hormone lowers serum calcium by releasing calcium from the bone

d. hypercalcemia (calcium levels greater than 10.2 mg/dl in adults and 10.7 mg/dl in children) is an indication for localizing abnormal parathyroid glands

16. When ultrasound fails to identify abnormal parathyroid glands preoperatively and postoperatively, the following tests are used

a. computed tomography, radionuclide scanning, or magnetic resonance imaging

b. arteriography and magnetic resonance imaging

c. computed tomography and spine radiography

d. none of the above

17. High resolution sonography recommended for the evaluation of parathyroid adenomas is between

a. 3.5 and 5.0 Mhz

b. 5.0 Mhz only

c. 7.5 and 10.0 Mhz

d. 2.5 Mhz only

18. Superior and inferior parathyroid glands are supplied

a. by superior thyroid arteries only

b. by both superior and inferior thyroid arteries

c. by the venous plexus only

d. by all of the above

Identify the structures indicated in the following illustrations. These figures duplicate those found in **ULTRASONOGRAPHY: Introduction to Normal Structure and Functional Anatomy**. Refer to the textbook if you need help.

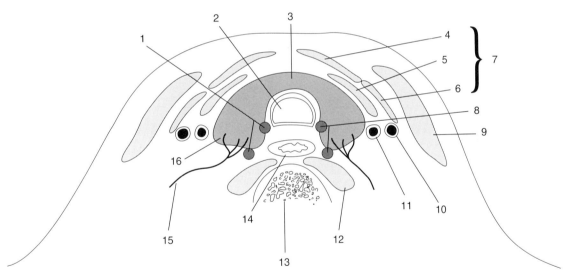

Figure 19–1. Thyroid anatomy and adjacent structures, transverse section.

1 _____

2 _____

3 _____

4 _____

5 _____

6 _____

7 _____

8 _____

9 _____

10 _____

11 _____

12 _____

13 _____

14 _____

15 _____

16 _____

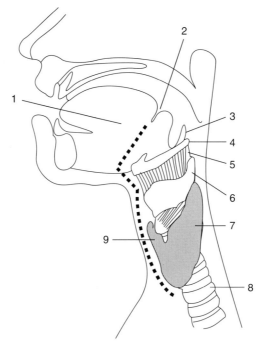

Figure 19-2. Embryonic migration of the thyroid gland. Broken line indicates path of migration.

1 _____   6 _____

2 _____   7 _____

3 _____   8 _____

4 _____   9 _____

5 _____

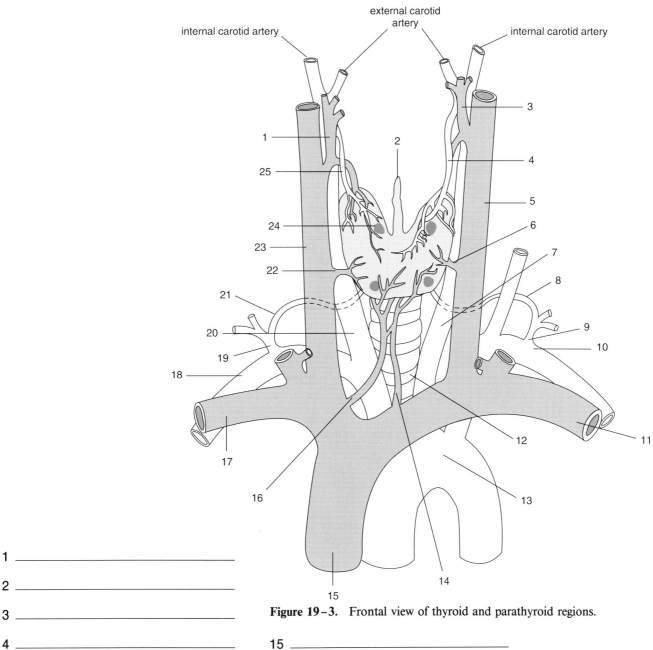

external carotid
artery

internal carotid artery

internal carotid artery

1

25

24

23

22

21

20

19

18

17

16

2

3

4

5

6

7

8

9

10

12

11

13

14

15

Figure 19-3. Frontal view of thyroid and parathyroid regions.

1 _____

2 _____

3 _____

4 _____

5 _____

6 _____

7 _____

8 _____

9 _____

10 _____

11 _____

12 _____

13 _____

14 _____

15 _____

16 _____

17 _____

18 _____

19 _____

20 _____

21 _____

22 _____

23 _____

24 _____

25 _____

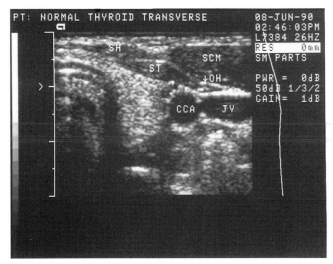 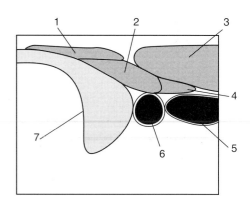

Figure 19-8. Thyroid gland and adjacent structures, transverse section.

1 _____   5 _____

2 _____   6 _____

3 _____   7 _____

4 _____

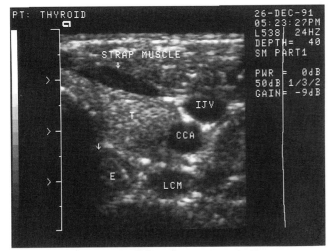 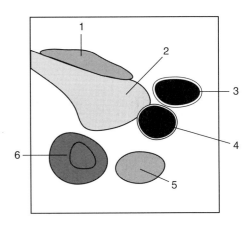

Figure 19-9. Thyroid gland and adjacent structures, transverse section.

1 _____   4 _____

2 _____   5 _____

3 _____   6 _____

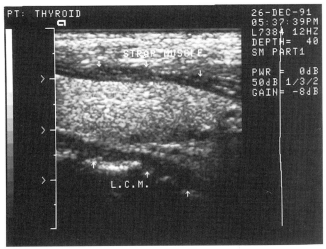 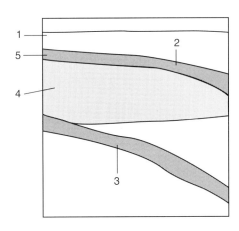

Figure 19-10. Thyroid gland and adjacent structures, sagittal section.

1 _____   4 _____

2 _____   5 _____

3 _____

1 _____

2 _____

3 _____

4 _____

5 _____

6 _____

7 _____

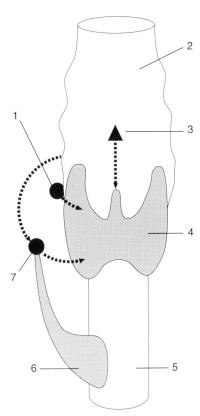

Figure 19-11. Migration of the thymus and parathyroid glands.

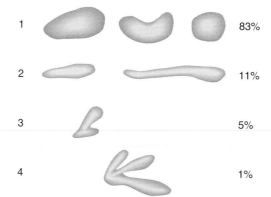

Figure 19–12. Parathyroid gland variations.

1 _____   3 _____

2 _____   4 _____

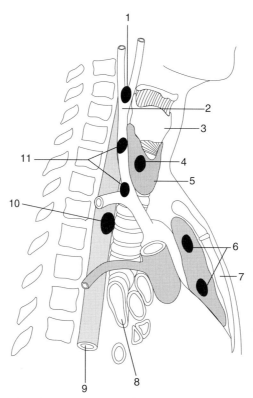

Figure 19–13. Aberrant locations of parathyroid glands.

1 _____   7 _____

2 _____   8 _____

3 _____   9 _____

4 _____   10 _____

5 _____   11 _____

6 _____

Chapter 20

THE BREAST

REVIEW QUESTIONS

1. Which of the following hormones does *not* affect the breast?

a. prolactin

b. progesterone

c. alkaline phosphatase

d. estrogen

2. Which of the following best describes the image shown?

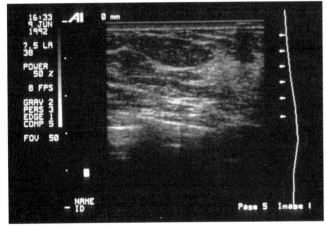

Image courtesy of Acoustic Imaging, Inc., Phoenix, AZ.

a. normal breast tissue

b. fatty breast tissue

c. fibrocystic breast changes

d. breast mass

e. breast cyst

3. Which of the following best describes the image shown?

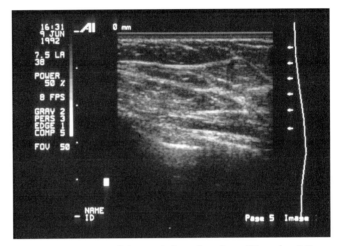

Image courtesy of Acoustic Imaging, Inc., Phoenix, AZ.

a. normal breast tissue

b. fatty breast tissue

c. fibrocystic breast changes

d. breast mass

e. breast cyst

4. Which of the following best describes the image shown?

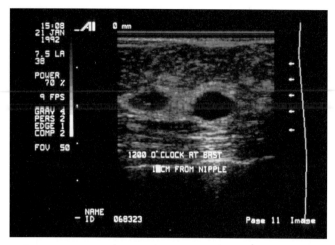

Image courtesy of Acoustic Imaging, Inc., Phoenix, AZ.

a. normal breast tissue

b. fatty breast tissue

c. fibrocystic breast changes

d. breast mass

e. breast cyst

5. The breast arises from which embryonic layer?

a. endoderm

b. mesoderm

c. mesenchyme

d. ectoderm

6. Which of the following best describes the image shown?

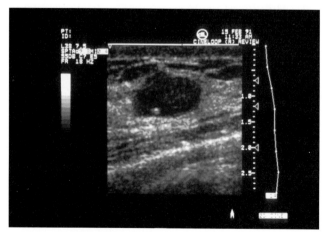

Image courtesy of Acoustic Imaging, Inc., Phoenix, AZ.

a. normal breast tissue

b. fatty breast tissue

c. fibrocystic breast changes

d. breast mass

e. breast cyst

7. Support of the breast parenchyma is provided by

a. lactiferous ducts

b. acini

c. Cooper's ligaments

d. the pectoralis major muscle

8. Which of the following statements best describes the anatomical location of the breast?

a. anterior to the pectoralis major muscle, bordered inferiorly by the fifth and sixth costal cartilages

b. anterior to the pectoralis major muscle, bordered superiorly by the second and third ribs

c. medial to the sternum, anterior to the second rib

d. anterior to the serratus muscle, lateral to the margin of the axilla

9. Most lymph drainage from the breast occurs in which manner?

a. subcutaneously

b. through the thoracic lymph nodes

c. through the acini

d. through the axillary lymph nodes

10. Which of the following statements is (are) true?

a. mammary glands are modified sweat glands

b. mammary glands are endocrine glands

c. mammary glands arise from the ectoderm

d. all of the above are true

Identify the structures indicated in the following illustrations. These figures duplicate those found in **ULTRASONOGRAPHY: Introduction to Normal Structure and Functional Anatomy**. Refer to the textbook if you need help.

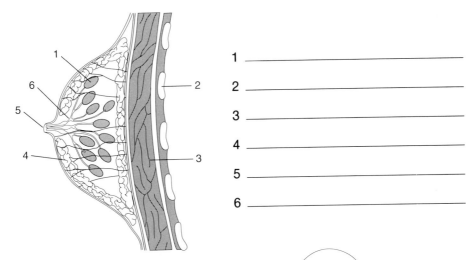

Figure 20–1. Cross section of breast anatomy.

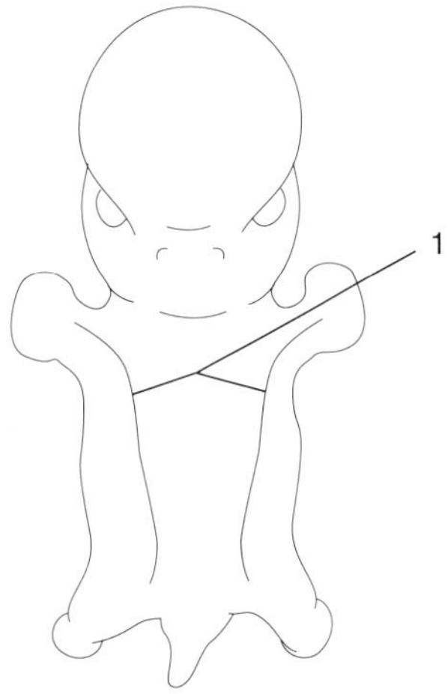

1 _____

2 _____

3 _____

4 _____

5 _____

6 _____

1 _____

Figure 20–2. Prenatal development of fetus.

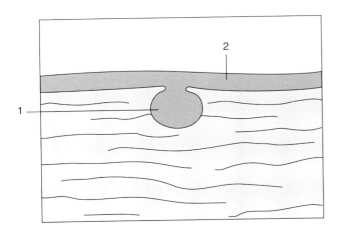

Connective tissue bud, 10 week gestation.

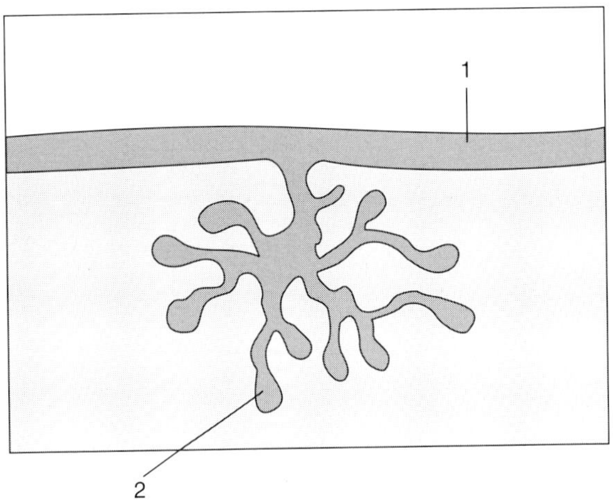

1 _____

2 _____

Lactiferous ducts, 4 month gestation.

1 _____

2 _____

Figure 20–3.

Image courtesy of Acoustic Imaging, Inc., Phoenix, AZ.

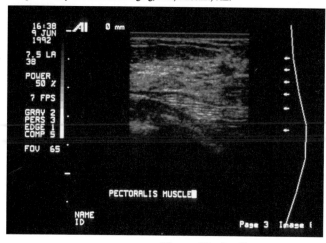
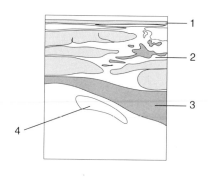

Figure 20–4. Breast anatomy and pectoralis muscle.

1 _____   3 _____

2 _____   4 _____

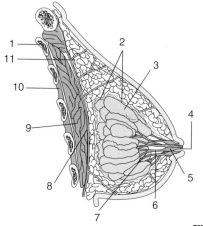
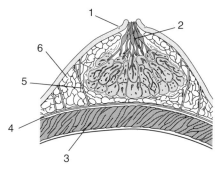

Figure 20–5. Breast anatomy.

1 _____   1 _____

2 _____   2 _____

3 _____   3 _____

4 _____   4 _____

5 _____   5 _____

6 _____   6 _____

7 _____

8 _____

9 _____

10 _____

11 _____

Image courtesy of Acoustic Imaging, Inc., Phoenix, AZ.

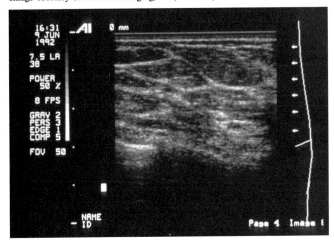 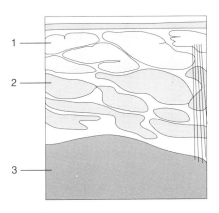

Figure 20-6. Anatomic layers of the breast.

1 _____

2 _____

3 _____

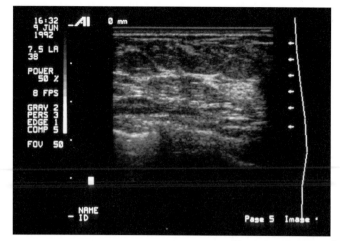
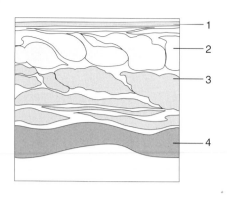

Fatty component of the breast.

1 _____ 3 _____

2 _____ 4 _____

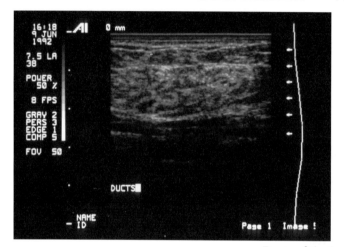
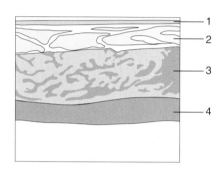

Ducts of the breast.

1 _____ 3 _____

2 _____ 4 _____

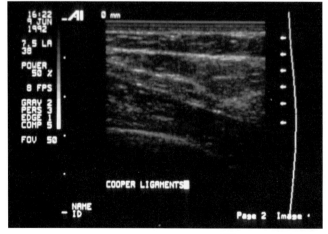
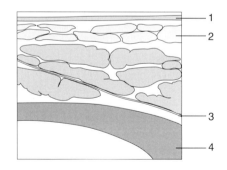

Fibrous component of the breast.

1 _____ 3 _____

2 _____ 4 _____

Figure 20-7.

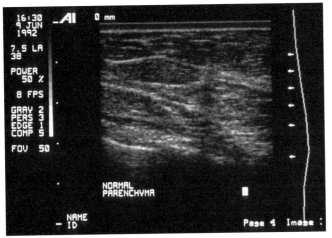 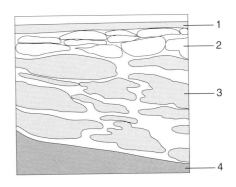

Glandular components of the breast.

1 _____   3 _____

2 _____   4 _____

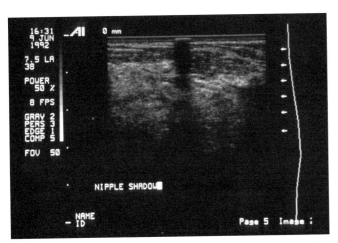 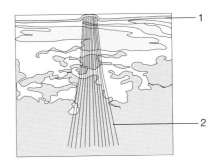

Nipple shadow.

1 _____

2 _____

Figure 20-7. *Continued*

All images in Figure 20-7 courtesy of Acoustic Imaging, Inc., Phoenix, AZ.

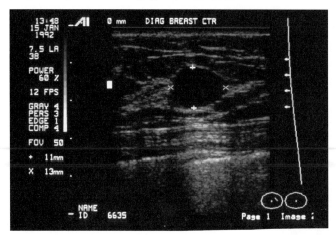 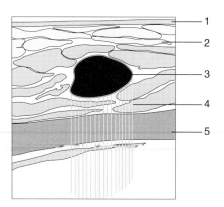

Breast cyst.

1 _____   4 _____

2 _____   5 _____

3 _____

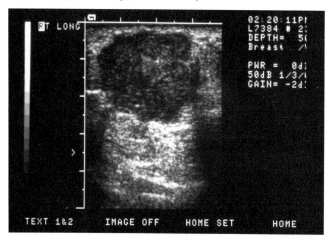

Solid breast mass.

1 _____

2 _____

3 _____

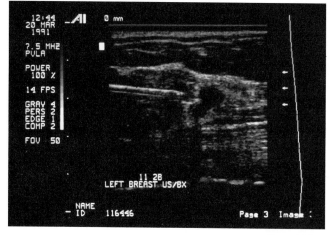 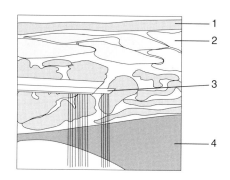

Breast biopsy.

1 _____   3 _____

2 _____   4 _____

Figure 20-8.

Image courtesy of Acoustic Imaging, Inc., Phoenix, AZ.

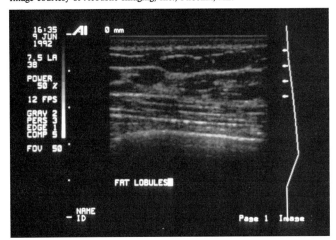
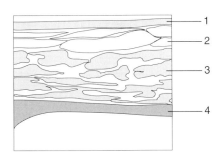

Fatty breast.

1 _____   3 _____

2 _____   4 _____

Image courtesy of DePaul Medical Center, Norfolk, VA.

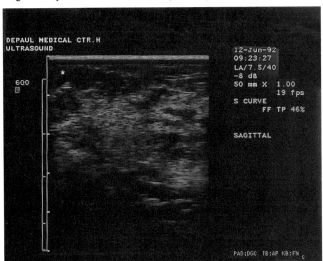
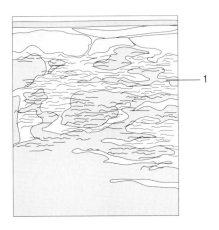

Fibrous breast.

1 _____

Figure 20–9.

Chapter 21

THE NEONATAL BRAIN

REVIEW QUESTIONS

1. Sonographically, the cisterna magna appears as an

a. anechoic space inferior to the cerebellum

b. anechoic space superior to the cerebellum

c. echogenic space inferior to the cerebellum

d. echogenic space superior to the cerebellum

2. The channel that connects the third and fourth ventricles is called

a. foramen of Luschka

b. foramen of Magendie

c. aqueduct of Sylvius

d. foramen of Monro

3. The moderately echogenic structure that marks the inferior and lateral margins of the frontal horns of the lateral ventricles is the

a. choroid plexus

b. massa intermedia

c. cavum septum pellucidum

d. head of the caudate nucleus

4. Located between the frontal horns of the lateral ventricles, and lying superior and anterior to the third ventricle, this midline, fluid-filled structure (ie, anechoic) is considered a normal variant

a. corpus callosum

b. foramen of Monro

c. cavum septum pellucidum

d. cavum velum interpositum

5. Anatomically, which vessels lie within the lateral sylvian fissures and are frequently seen pulsating during a real-time examination?

a. anterior cerebral arteries

b. middle cerebral arteries

c. posterior cerebral arteries

d. basilar arteries

6. Which of the following best describes the position of the choroid plexus within the ventricles? It is located within

a. the occipital horns of the lateral ventricles only

b. the frontal, occipital, and temporal horns and bodies of the lateral ventricles only

c. the roof of the third and fourth ventricles only

d. the trigone region of the lateral ventricles, the medial aspects of the temporal horns, and the roof of both the third and fourth ventricles

7. Which of the following structures is *not* sonographically echogenic?

a. fourth ventricle

b. cerebellar vermis

c. choroid plexus

d. quadrigeminal plate cistern

258

Identify the structures indicated in the following illustrations. These figures duplicate those found in **ULTRASONOGRAPHY: Introduction to Normal Structure and Functional Anatomy**. Refer to the textbook if you need help.

Images redrawn from Tempkin BB: Ultrasound Scanning: Principles and Protocols. Philadelphia, WB Saunders, 1993, p. 238.

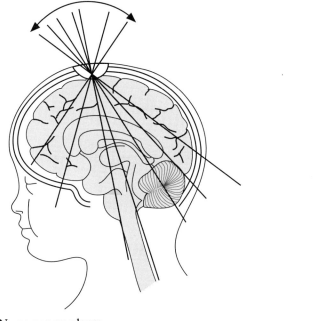

Name survey plane: _____

Figure 21–1.

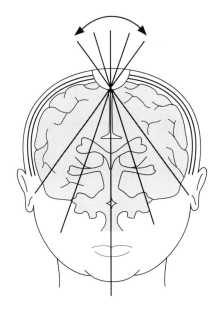

Name survey plane: _____

Figure 21–2.

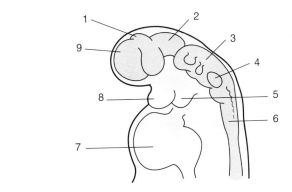

1 _____   6 _____

2 _____   7 _____

3 _____   8 _____

4 _____   9 _____

5 _____

Figure 21–3. 3½ weeks brain development.

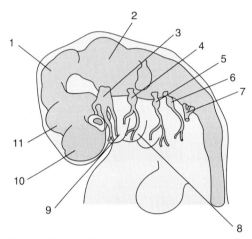

Figure 21–4. 5½ weeks brain development.

1 _____		7 _____		
2 _____		8 _____		
3 _____		9 _____		
4 _____		10 _____		
5 _____		11 _____		
6 _____				

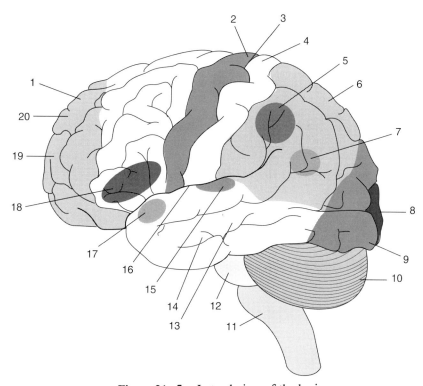

Figure 21–5. Lateral view of the brain.

1 _____

2 _____

3 _____

4 _____

5 _____

6 _____

7 _____

8 _____

9 _____

10 _____

11 _____

12 _____

13 _____

14 _____

15 _____

16 _____

17 _____

18 _____

19 _____

20 _____

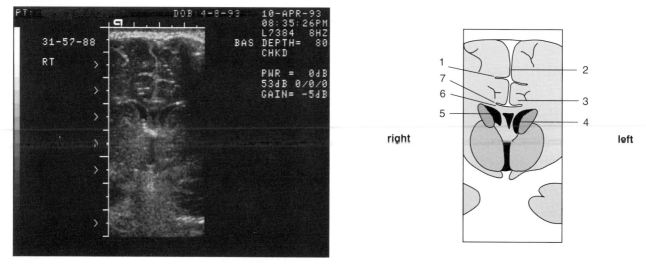

Figure 21-6. Brain coronal section.

1 _____   5 _____

2 _____   6 _____

3 _____   7 _____

4 _____

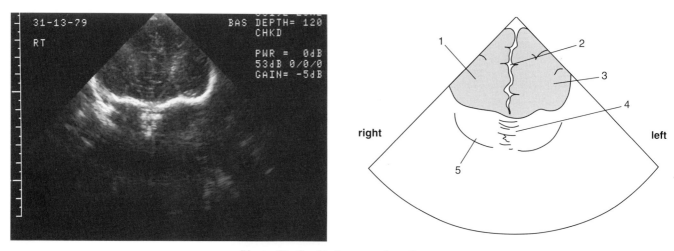

Figure 21-7. Brain coronal section.

1 _____   4 _____

2 _____   5 _____

3 _____

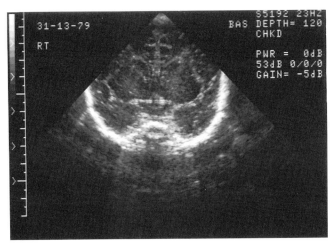
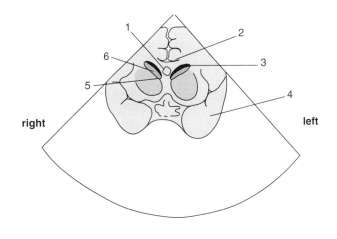

Figure 21–8. Brain coronal section.

1 _____ 4 _____

2 _____ 5 _____

3 _____ 6 _____

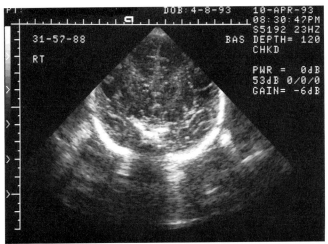
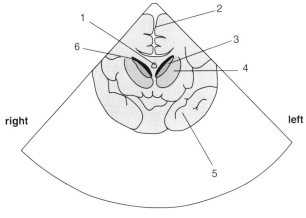

Figure 21–9. Brain coronal section.

1 _____ 4 _____

2 _____ 5 _____

3 _____ 6 _____

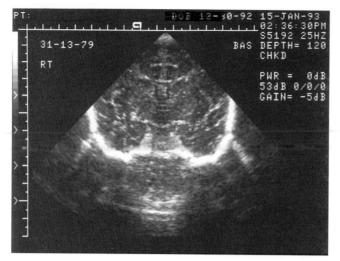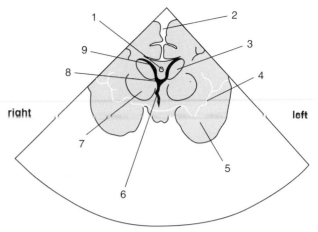

Figure 21–10. Brain coronal section.

1 _____   6 _____

2 _____   7 _____

3 _____   8 _____

4 _____   9 _____

5 _____

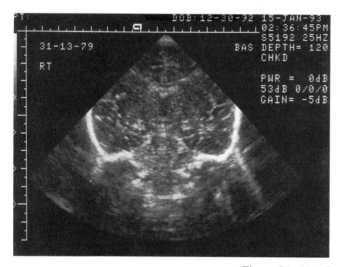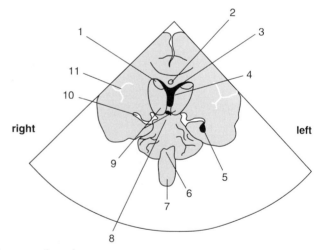

Figure 21–11. Brain coronal section.

1 _____   7 _____

2 _____   8 _____

3 _____   9 _____

4 _____   10 _____

5 _____   11 _____

6 _____

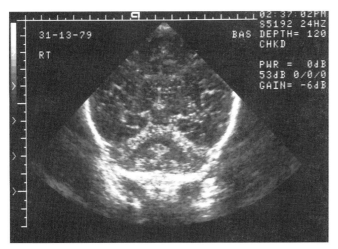 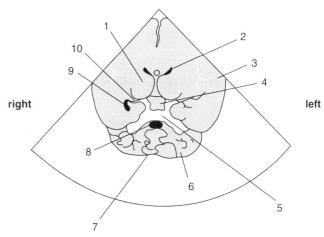

Figure 21–12. Brain coronal section.

1 _____	6 _____
2 _____	7 _____
3 _____	8 _____
4 _____	9 _____
5 _____	10 _____

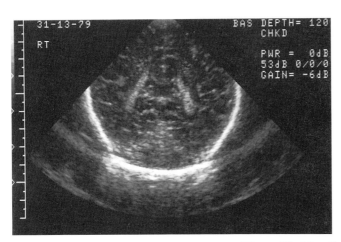 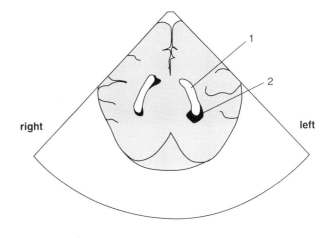

Figure 21–13. Brain coronal section.

1 _____

2 _____

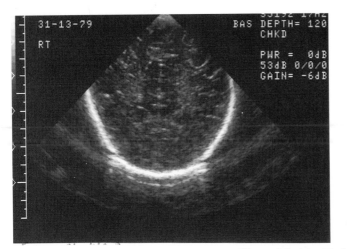
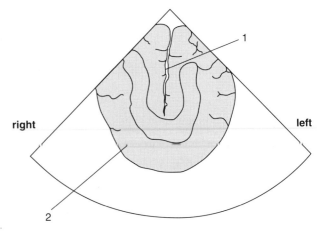

Figure 21–14. Brain coronal section.

1 _____

2 _____

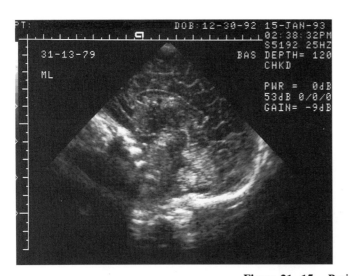
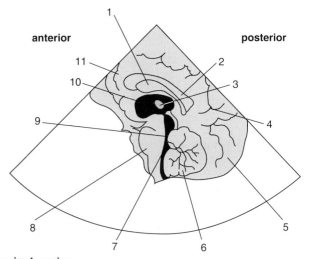

Figure 21–15. Brain sagittal section.

1 _____	7 _____
2 _____	8 _____
3 _____	9 _____
4 _____	10 _____
5 _____	11 _____
6 _____	

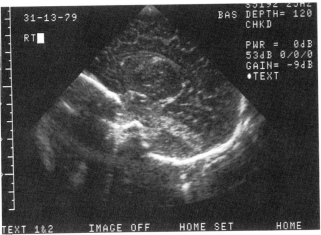 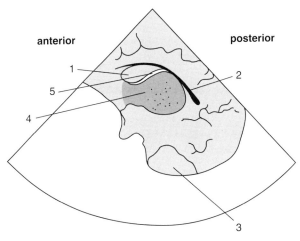

Figure 21–16. Brain sagittal section.

1 _____   4 _____

2 _____   5 _____

3 _____

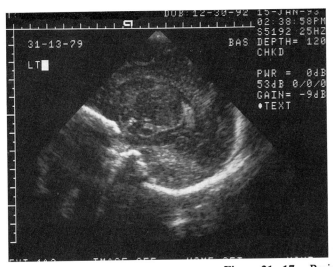 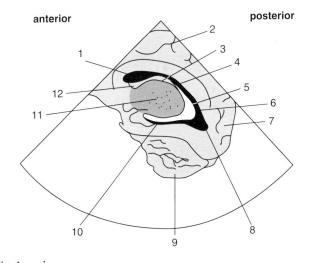

Figure 21–17. Brain sagittal section.

1 _____   7 _____

2 _____   8 _____

3 _____   9 _____

4 _____   10 _____

5 _____   11 _____

6 _____   12 _____

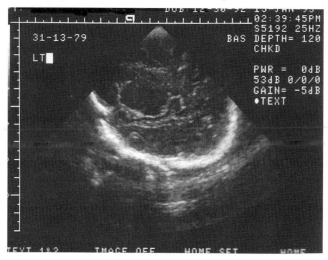 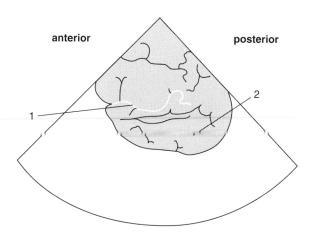

Figure 21–18. Brain sagittal section.

1 _____

2 _____

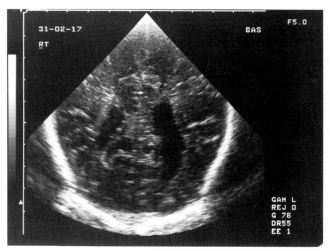 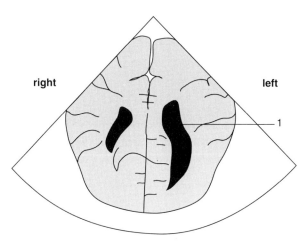

Figure 21–19. Brain coronal section.

1 _____

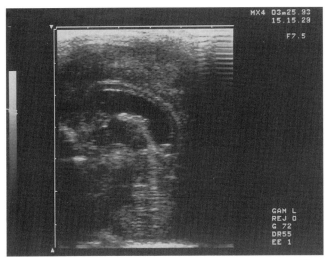
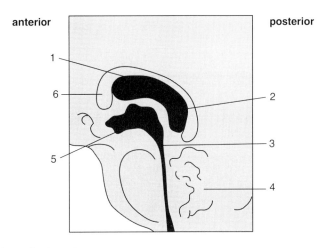

Figure 21–20. Brain sagittal section.

1 _____   4 _____

2 _____   5 _____

3 _____   6 _____

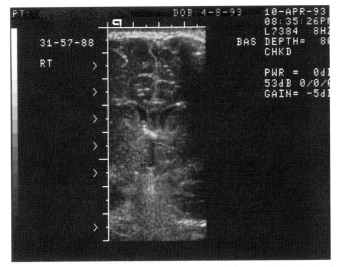
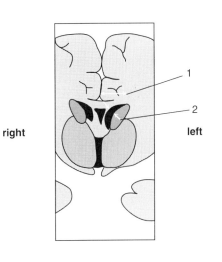

Figure 21–21. Brain coronal section.

1 _____

2 _____

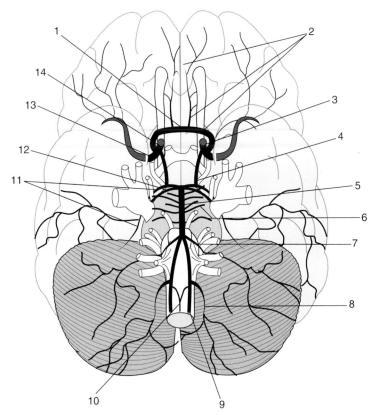

Figure 21-22. Brain arterial supply.

1 _____
2 _____
3 _____
4 _____
5 _____
6 _____
7 _____
8 _____
9 _____
10 _____
11 _____
12 _____
13 _____
14 _____

1 _____
2 _____
3 _____
4 _____
5 _____
6 _____
7 _____
8 _____
9 _____
10 _____
11 _____
12 _____

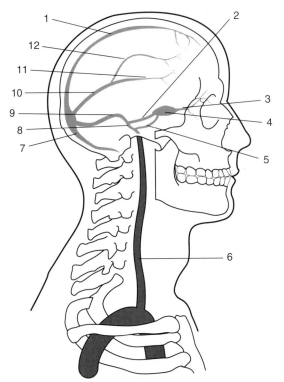

Figure 21-23. Major venous drainage of the brain.

Chapter 22

PEDIATRIC ECHOCARDIOGRAPHY

REVIEW QUESTIONS

1. Describe the function of the heart.

2. Describe the location of the heart and the surrounding structures.

3. Describe blood flow through the heart.

4. What is defined as the pulmonary circulation?

5. What is defined as the systemic circulation?

6. Describe the parts of the heart and their sonographic appearance.

7. Describe the cardiac conduction system.

8. Briefly describe cardiac perfusion and drainage.

9. Which physician specializes in managing diseases of the heart?

10. Name two diagnostic tests of the heart and the personnel who perform and interpret these tests.

11. Describe the relative differences in oxygen content and pressures between the right heart and the left heart.

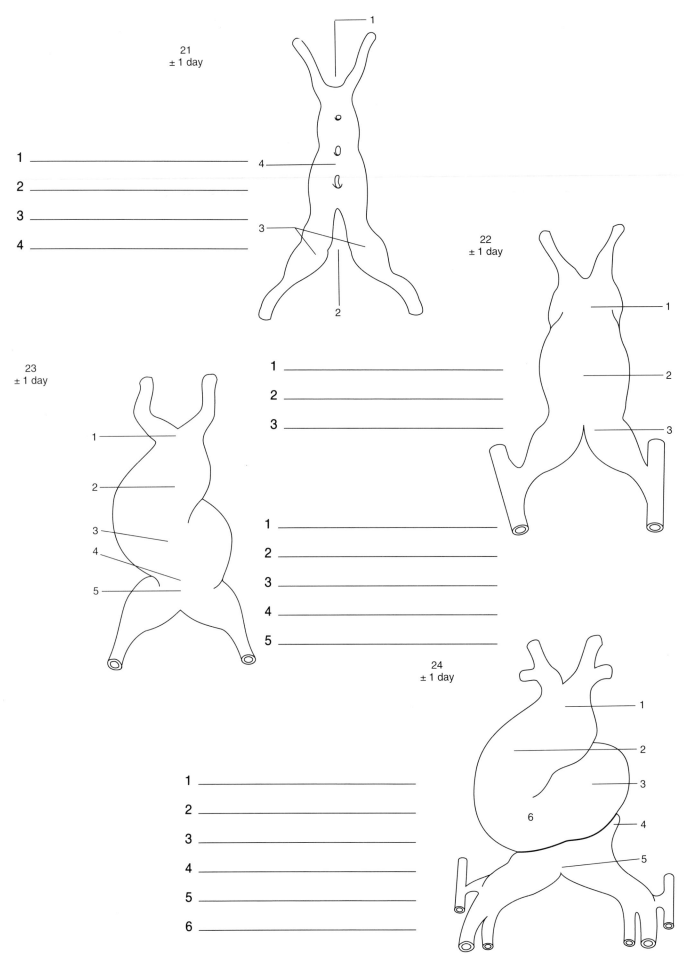

Figure 22-1. Ventral views of developing heart at 20 to 25 days.

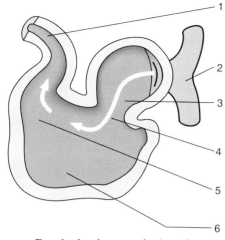

Developing heart sagittal section.

1 _____

2 _____

3 _____

4 _____

5 _____

6 _____

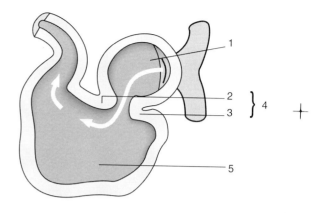

Developing heart sagittal section.

1 _____

2 _____

3 _____

4 _____

5 _____

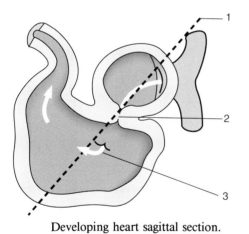

Developing heart sagittal section.

1 _____

2 _____

3 _____

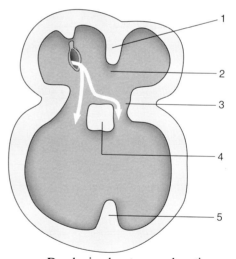

Developing heart coronal section.

1 _____

2 _____

3 _____

4 _____

5 _____

Figure 22–2.

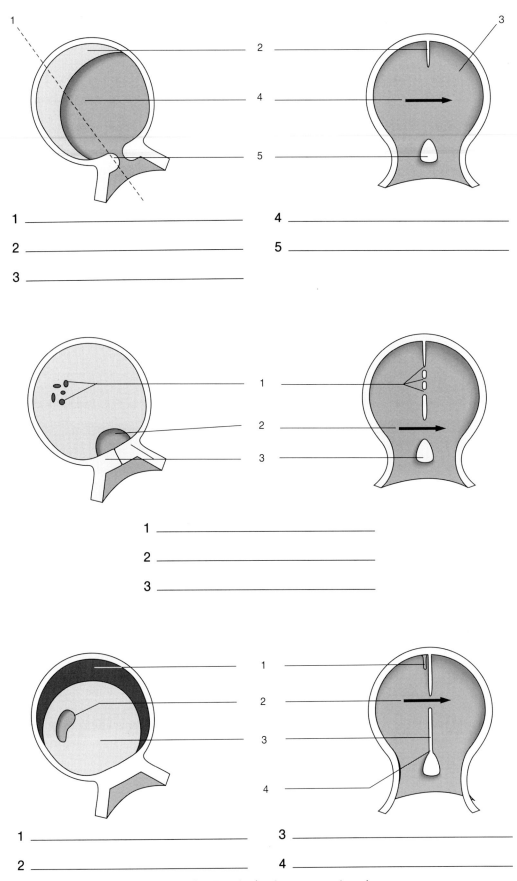

1 _____

2 _____

3 _____

4 _____

5 _____

1 _____

2 _____

3 _____

1 _____

2 _____

3 _____

4 _____

Figure 22–3. Developing heart coronal sections.

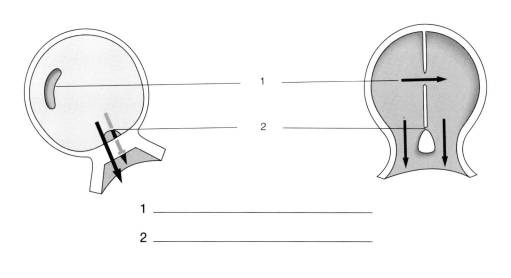

1 _____

2 _____

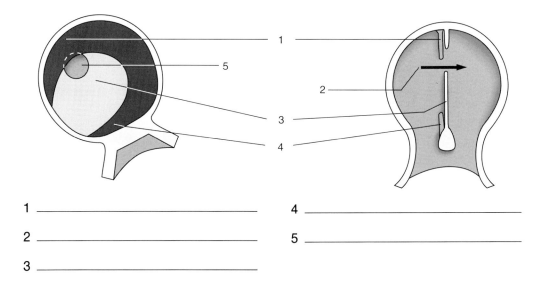

1 _____   4 _____

2 _____   5 _____

3 _____

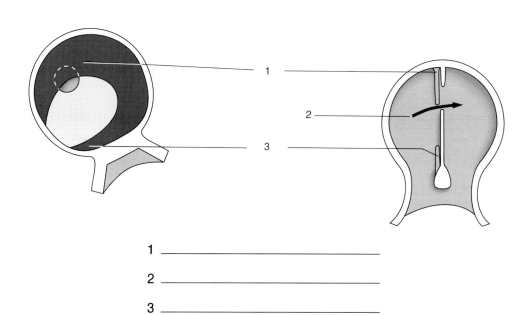

1 _____

2 _____

3 _____

Figure 22–3. *Continued*

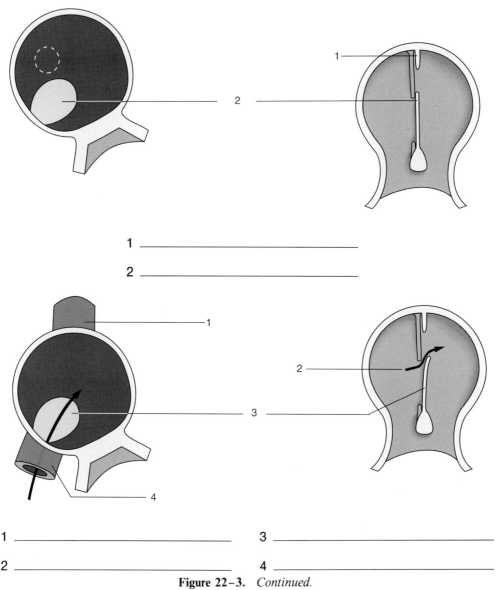

1 _____

2 _____

1 _____   3 _____

2 _____   4 _____

Figure 22–3. *Continued.*

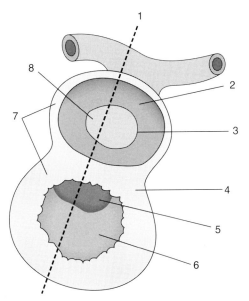

Developing heart, 5th week, sagittal section.

1 _____   5 _____

2 _____   6 _____

3 _____   7 _____

4 _____   8 _____

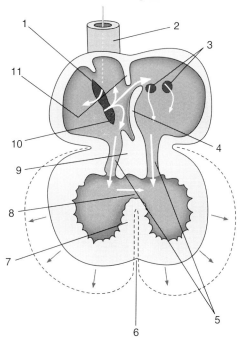

Developing heart coronal section.

1 _____   7 _____

2 _____   8 _____

3 _____   9 _____

4 _____   10 _____

5 _____   11 _____

6 _____

Figure 22–4.

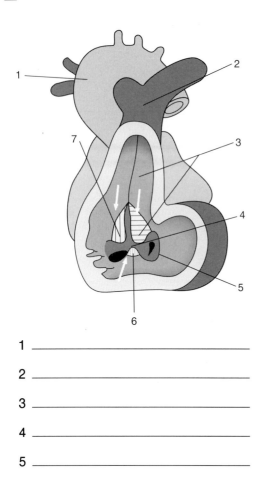

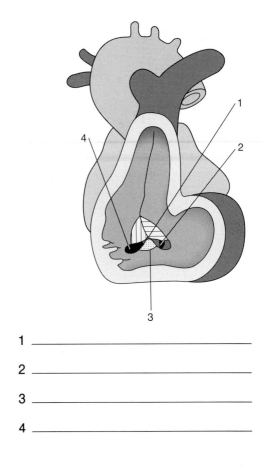

1 _____

2 _____

3 _____

4 _____

5 _____

6 _____

7 _____

1 _____

2 _____

3 _____

4 _____

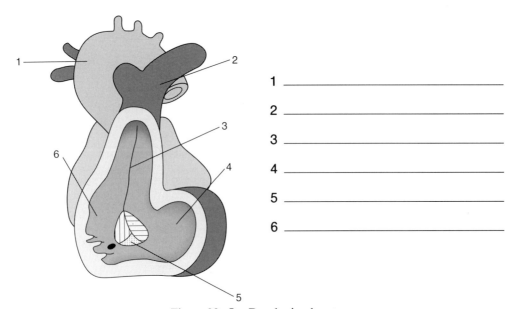

1 _____

2 _____

3 _____

4 _____

5 _____

6 _____

Figure 22–5. Developing heart.

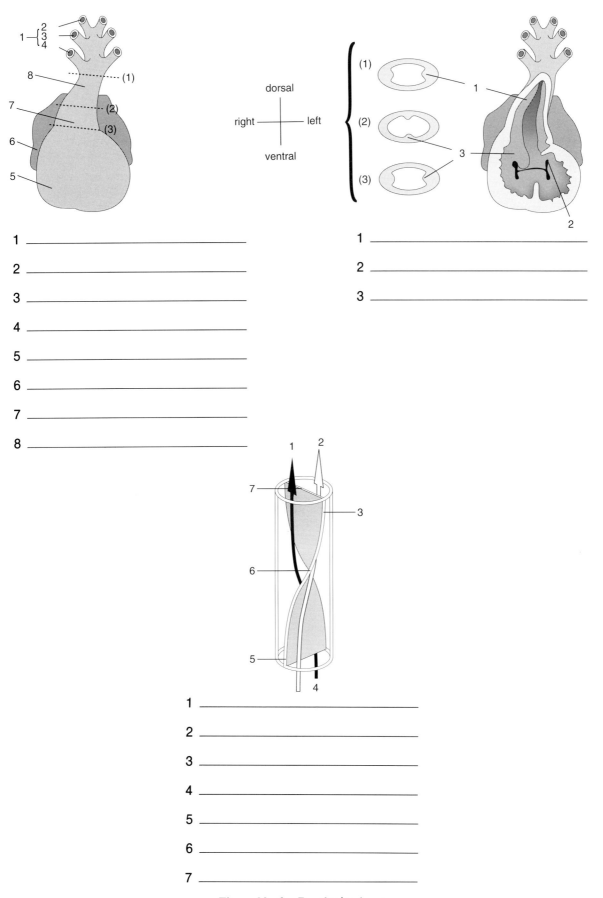

Figure 22-6. Developing heart.

1 _____

2 _____

3 _____

4 _____

5 _____

6 _____

7 _____

8 _____

1 _____

2 _____

3 _____

1 _____

2 _____

3 _____

4 _____

5 _____

6 _____

7 _____

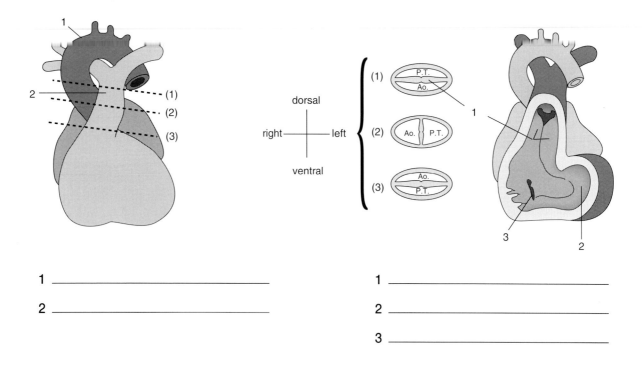

1 _____

2 _____

1 _____

2 _____

3 _____

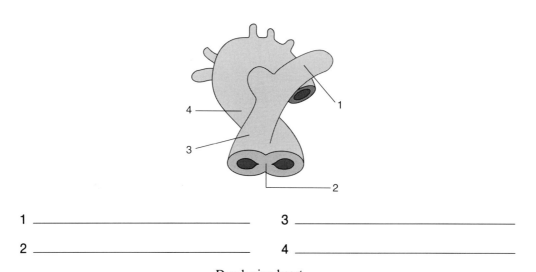

1 _____   3 _____

2 _____   4 _____

Developing heart.

Figure 22–6. *Continued*

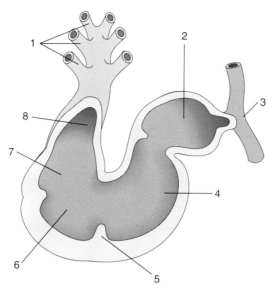

Developing heart, 5 weeks, sagittal section.

1 _____   5 _____

2 _____   6 _____

3 _____   7 _____

4 _____   8 _____

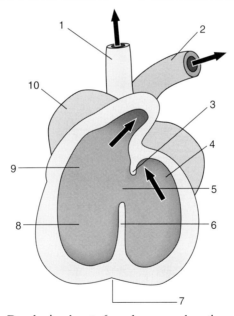

Developing heart, 6 weeks, coronal section.

1 _____   6 _____

2 _____   7 _____

3 _____   8 _____

4 _____   9 _____

5 _____   10 _____

Figure 22–7.

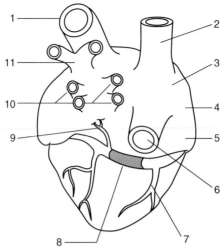

Figure 22–8. Developing heart, 8 weeks, dorsal view.

1 _____   7 _____

2 _____   8 _____

3 _____   9 _____

4 _____   10 _____

5 _____   11 _____

6 _____

---

 1 _____   15 _____

 2 _____   16 _____

 3 _____   17 _____

 4 _____   18 _____

 5 _____   19 _____

 6 _____   20 _____

 7 _____   21 _____

 8 _____   22 _____

 9 _____   23 _____

10 _____   24 _____

11 _____   25 _____

12 _____   26 _____

13 _____   27 _____

14 _____

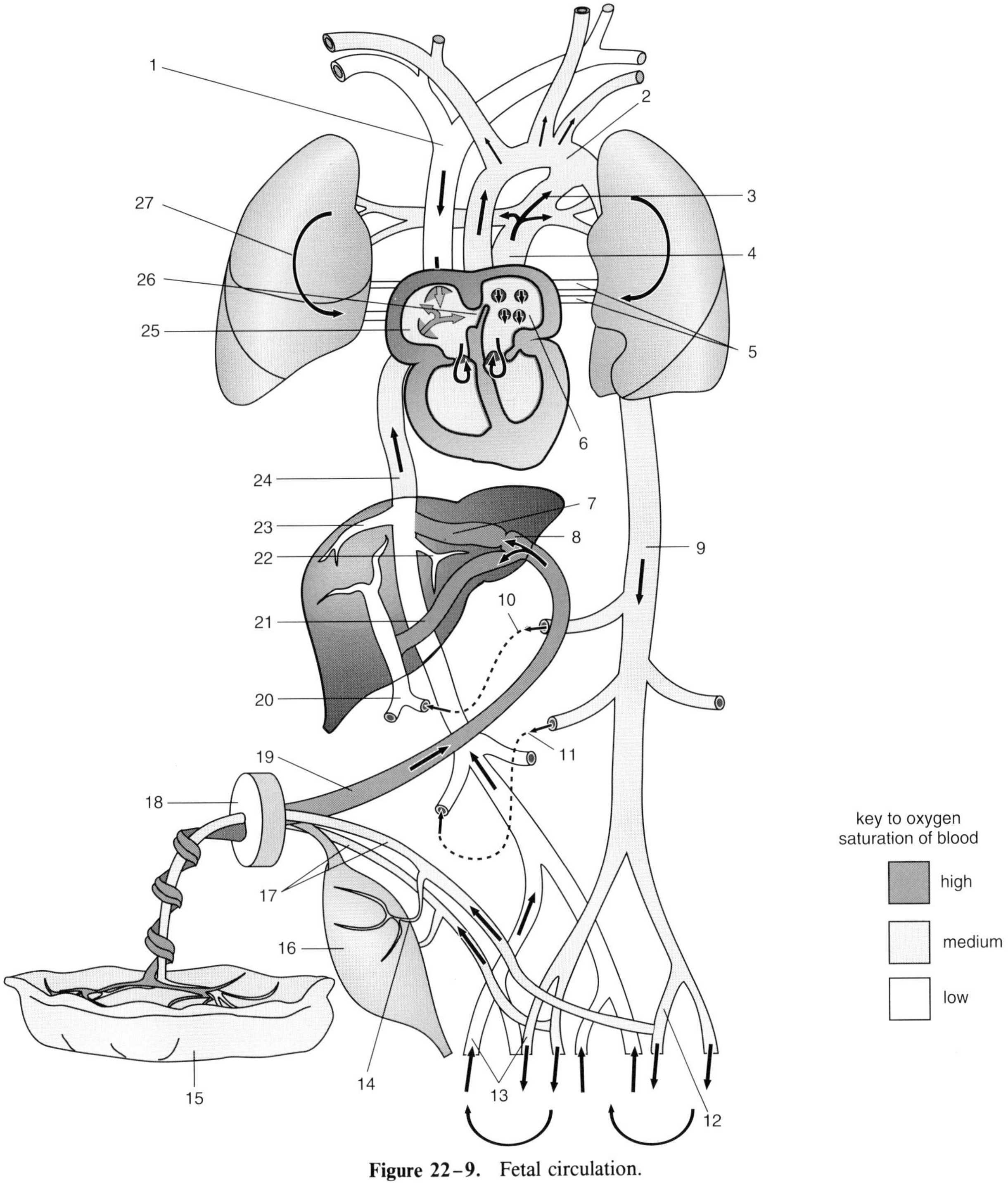

Figure 22–9. Fetal circulation.

key to oxygen
saturation of blood

high

medium

low

1 _____

2 _____

3 _____

4 _____

5 _____

6 _____

7 _____

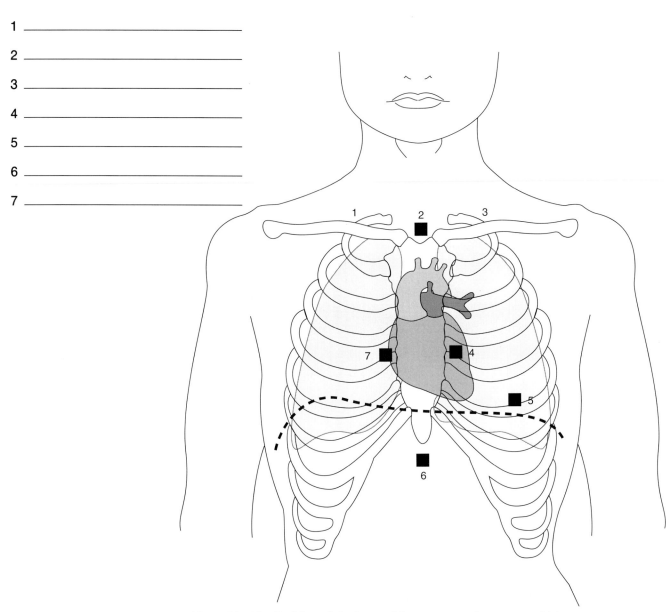

Figure 22–10. Position of the heart with respect to other organs within the chest cavity.

1 _____   9 _____

2 _____   10 _____

3 _____   11 _____

4 _____   12 _____

5 _____   13 _____

6 _____   14 _____

7 _____   15 _____

8 _____   16 _____

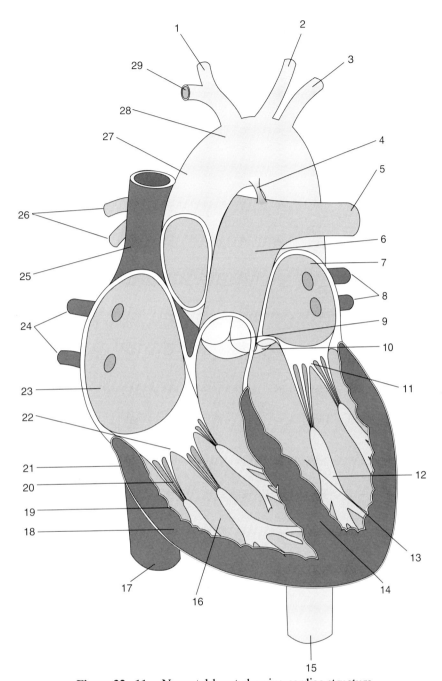

Figure 22–11. Neonatal heart showing cardiac structure.

17 _____   24 _____

18 _____   25 _____

19 _____   26 _____

20 _____   27 _____

21 _____   28 _____

22 _____   29 _____

23 _____

1 _____   13 _____

2 _____   14 _____

3 _____   15 _____

4 _____   16 _____

5 _____   17 _____

6 _____   18 _____

7 _____   19 _____

8 _____   20 _____

9 _____   21 _____

10 _____   22 _____

11 _____   23 _____

12 _____   24 _____

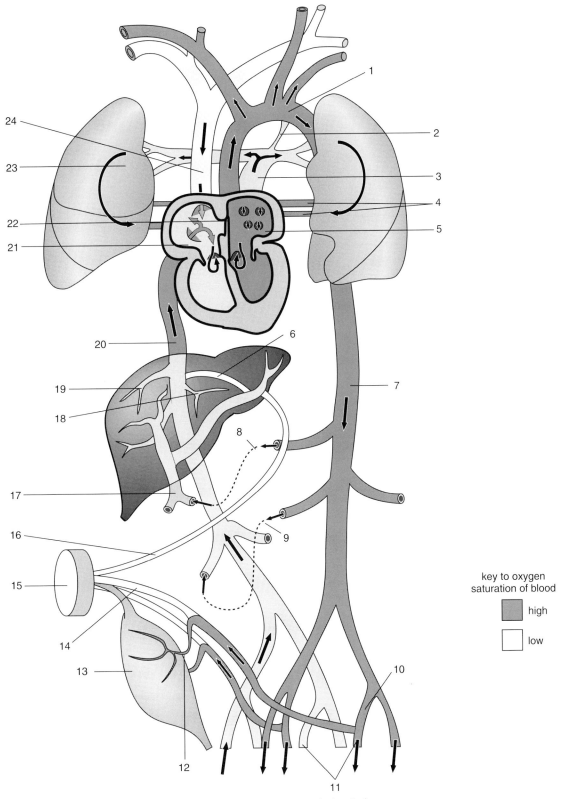

Figure 22–12. Neonatal circulation.

1 _____

2 _____

3 _____

4 _____

5 _____

6 _____

7 _____

8 _____

9 _____

10 _____

11 _____

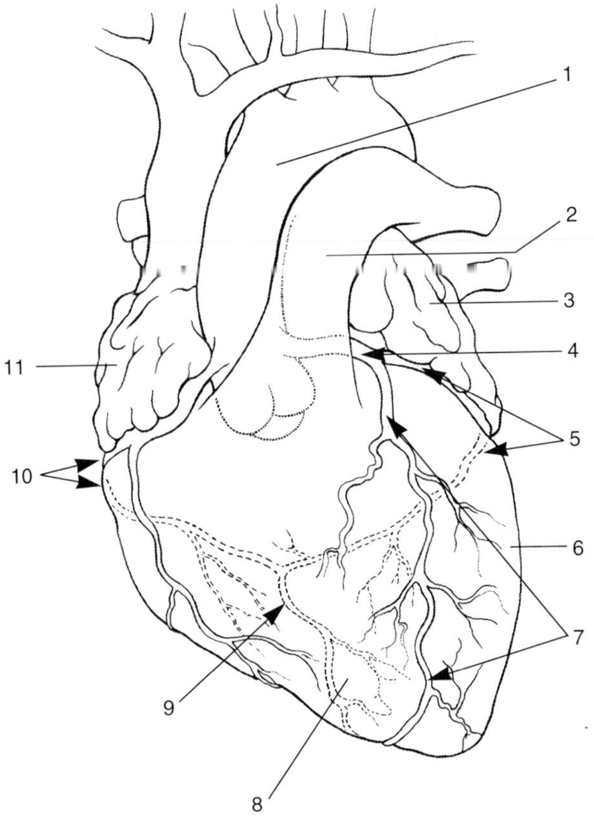

Coronary arteries and their positions on the heart, anterior view.

1 _____

2 _____

3 _____

4 _____

5 _____

6 _____

7 _____

8 _____

9 _____

10 _____

11 _____

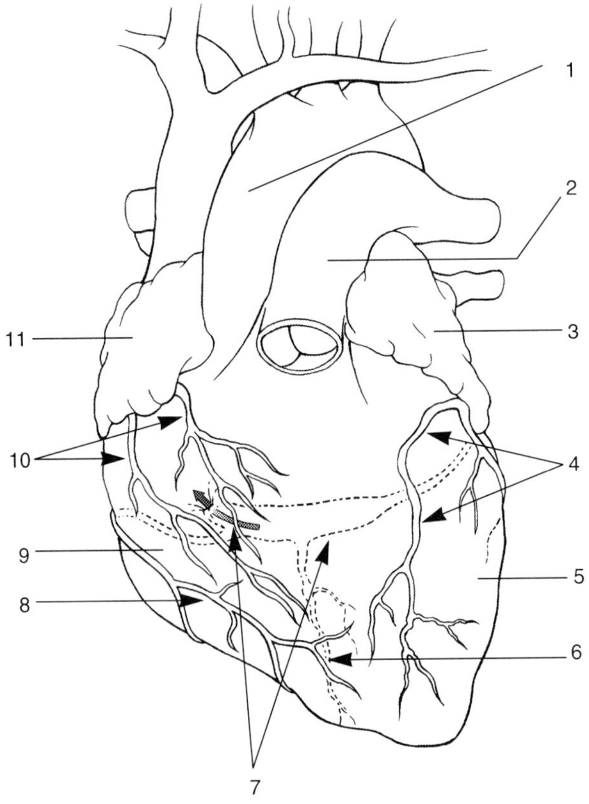

Cardiac veins and their positions on the heart, anterior view.

Figure 22–13.

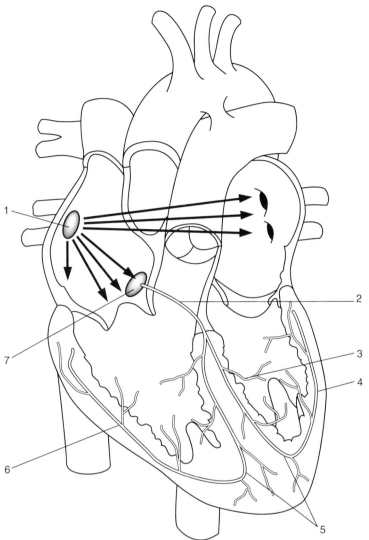

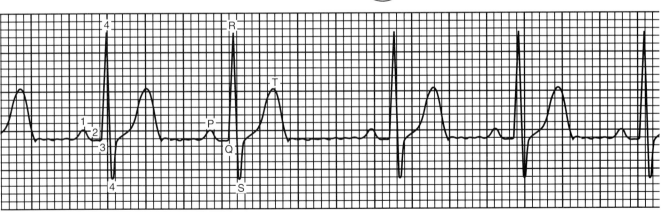

Figure 22–14. Cardiac conduction system.

1 _____   5 _____

2 _____   6 _____

3 _____   7 _____

4 _____

1 _____

2 _____

3 _____

4 _____

1 _____

2 _____

3 _____

4 _____

5 _____

6 _____

7 _____

1 _____

2 _____

3 _____

4 _____

5 _____

6 _____

7 _____

1 _____

2 _____

3 _____

1 _____

2 _____

3 _____

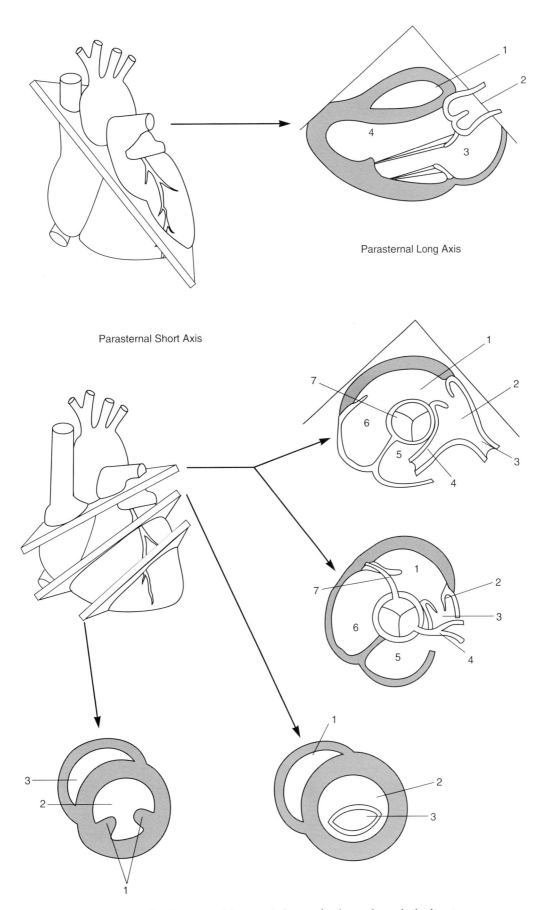

Parasternal Long Axis

Parasternal Short Axis

Figure 22–15. Parasternal long and short axis planes through the heart.

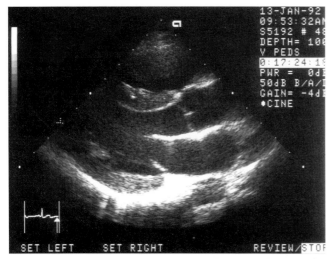
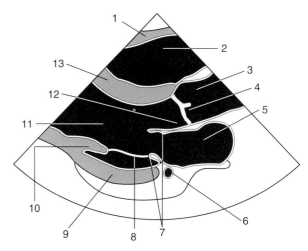

Parasternal long axis view, diastolic frame.

1 _____   8 _____

2 _____   9 _____

3 _____   10 _____

4 _____   11 _____

5 _____   12 _____

6 _____   13 _____

7 _____

Figure 22–16.

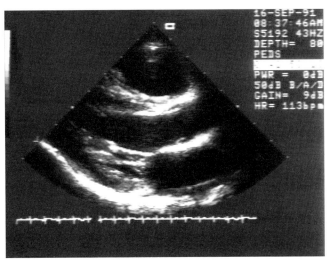
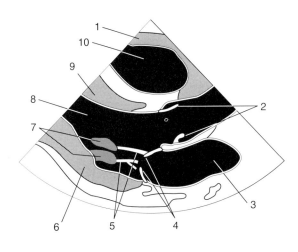

Parasternal long axis view, systolic frame.

1 _____	6 _____
2 _____	7 _____
3 _____	8 _____
4 _____	9 _____
5 _____	10 _____

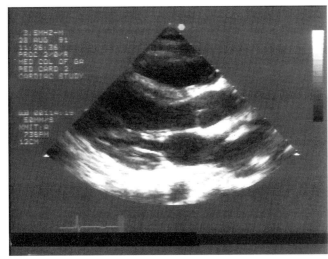
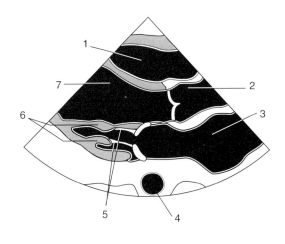

Parasternal long axis view, late diastolic frame.

1 _____	5 _____
2 _____	6 _____
3 _____	7 _____
4 _____	

Figure 22–16. *Continued*

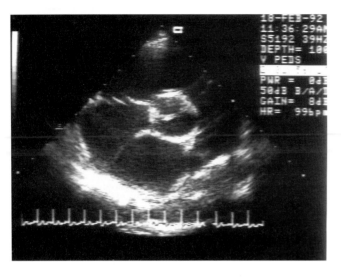
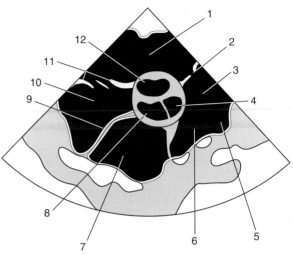

Closed aortic valve, parasternal short axis section.

1 _____   7 _____

2 _____   8 _____

3 _____   9 _____

4 _____   10 _____

5 _____   11 _____

6 _____   12 _____

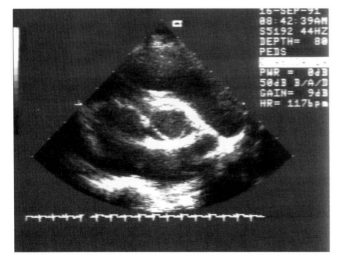
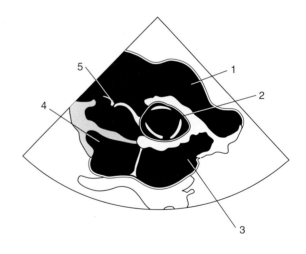

Open aortic valve, parasternal short axis section.

1 _____   4 _____

2 _____   5 _____

3 _____

Figure 22–21.

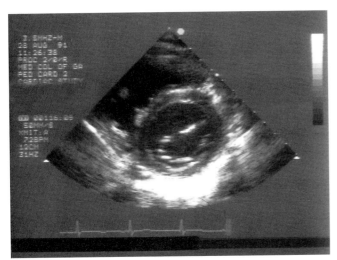
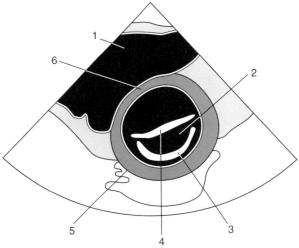

Mitral valve short axis plane.

1 _____   4 _____

2 _____   5 _____

3 _____   6 _____

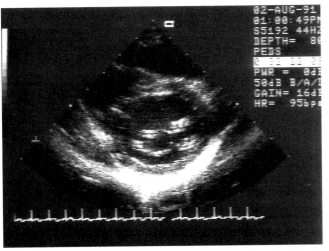
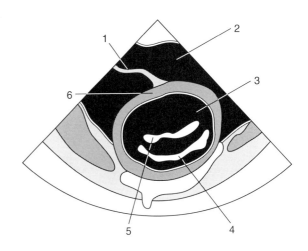

Mitral valve short axis plane.

1 _____   4 _____

2 _____   5 _____

3 _____   6 _____

Figure 22–22.

1 _____

2 _____

3 _____

4 _____

5 _____

6 _____

7 _____

8 _____

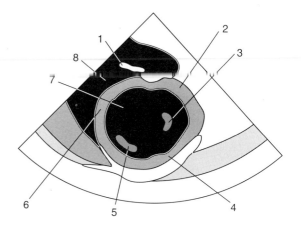

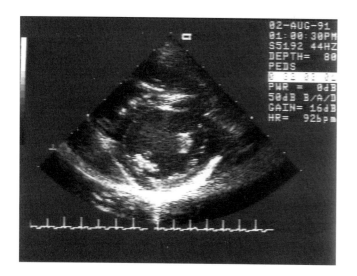

1 _____

2 _____

3 _____

4 _____

5 _____

6 _____

7 _____

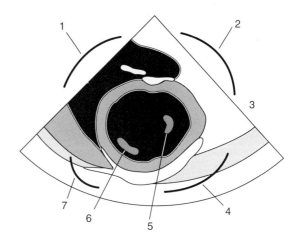

Figure 22–23. Left ventricle at papillary muscle level.

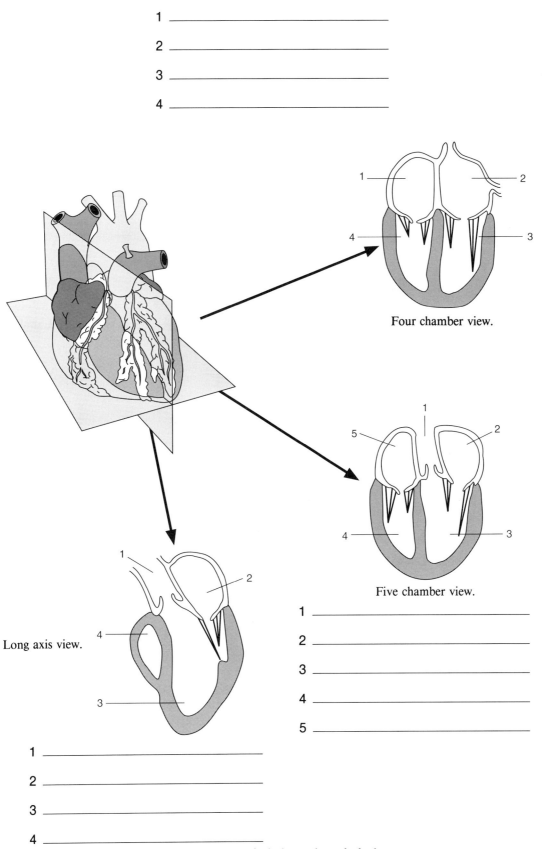

1 _____

2 _____

3 _____

4 _____

Four chamber view.

Five chamber view.

Long axis view.

1 _____

2 _____

3 _____

4 _____

5 _____

1 _____

2 _____

3 _____

4 _____

Figure 22–24. Apical planes through the heart.

From Park MK: Pediatric Cardiology for Practitioners. Chicago, Year Book, 1988.

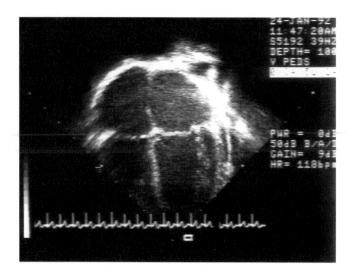
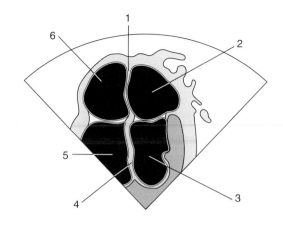

1 _____   4 _____

2 _____   5 _____

3 _____   6 _____

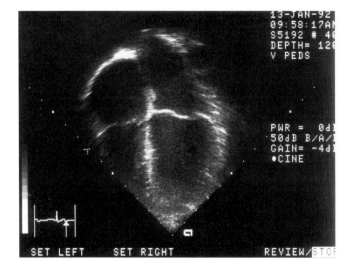
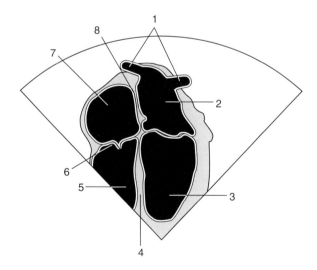

1 _____   5 _____

2 _____   6 _____

3 _____   7 _____

4 _____   8 _____

Figure 22-25. Apical four chamber sections.

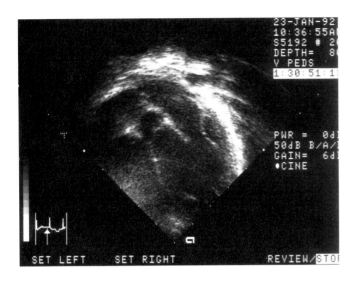
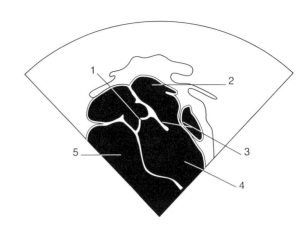

1 _____   4 _____

2 _____   5 _____

3 _____

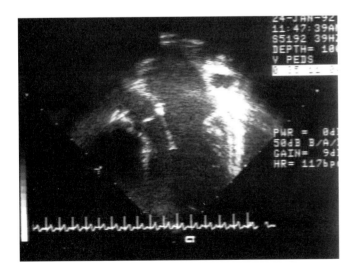
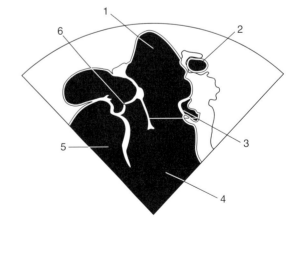

1 _____   4 _____

2 _____   5 _____

3 _____   6 _____

Figure 22-26. Apical long axis sections.

(Top right image)

1 _____

2 _____

3 _____

4 _____

5 _____

6 _____

(Middle right image)

1 _____

2 _____

3 _____

4 _____

5 _____

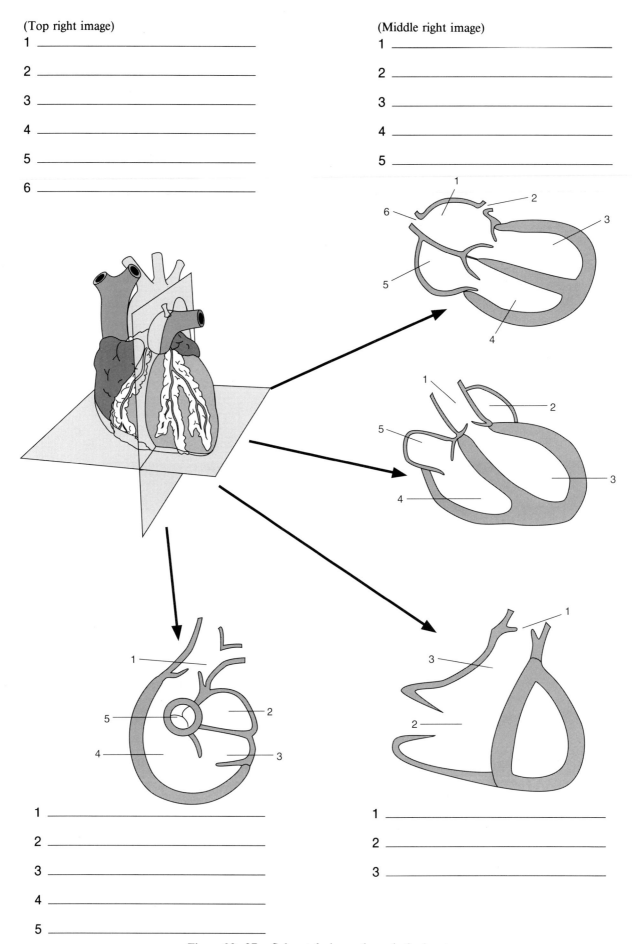

1 _____

2 _____

3 _____

4 _____

5 _____

1 _____

2 _____

3 _____

Figure 22–27. Subcostal planes through the heart.

300

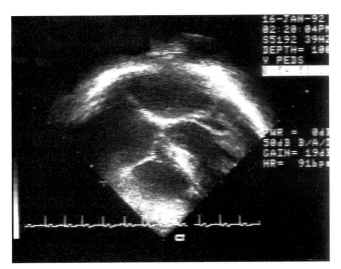
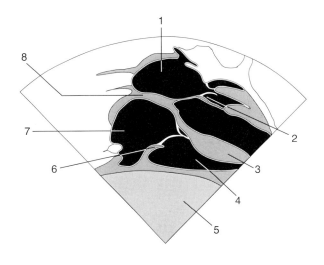

Figure 22–28. Subcostal four chamber section.

1 _____   5 _____

2 _____   6 _____

3 _____   7 _____

4 _____   8 _____

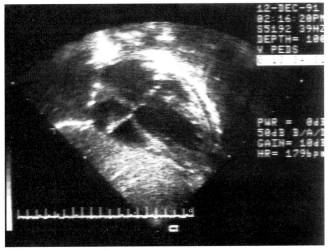
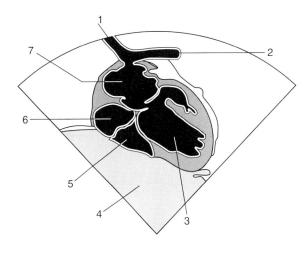

Figure 22–29. Subcostal four chamber section.

1 _____   5 _____

2 _____   6 _____

3 _____   7 _____

4 _____

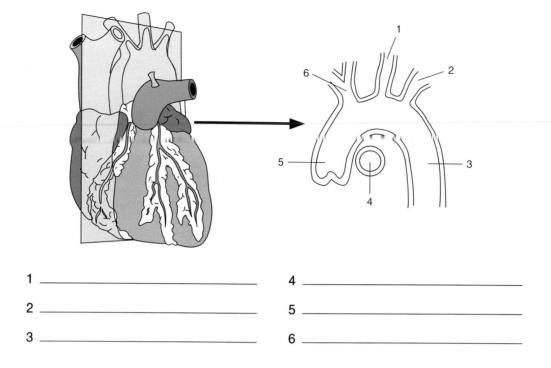

1 _____   4 _____

2 _____   5 _____

3 _____   6 _____

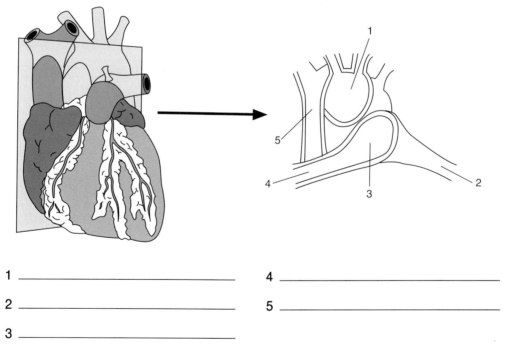

1 _____   4 _____

2 _____   5 _____

3 _____

Figure 22–30. Suprasternal planes through the heart.

From Park MK: Pediatric Cardiology for Practitioners. Chicago, Year Book, 1988.

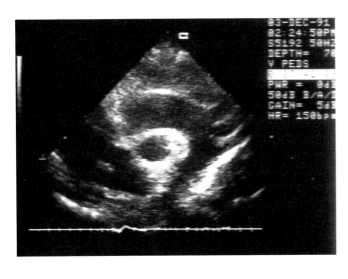
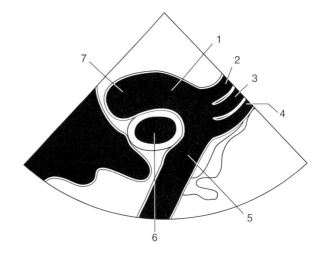

1 _____   5 _____

2 _____   6 _____

3 _____   7 _____

4 _____

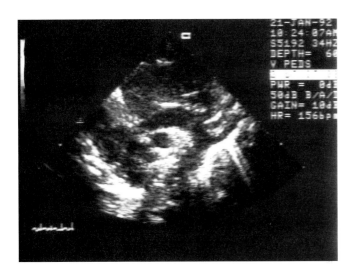
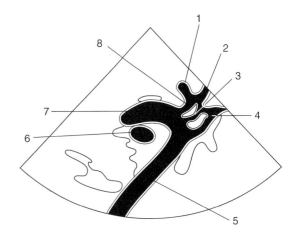

1 _____   5 _____

2 _____   6 _____

3 _____   7 _____

4 _____   8 _____

Figure 22–31. Aortic arch long axis.

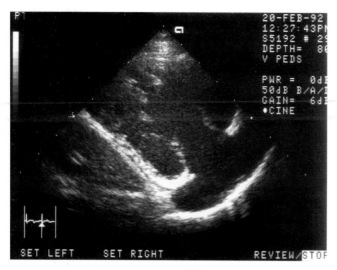
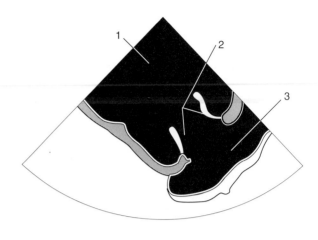

Right ventricular inflow tract, long axis, diastolic image.

1 _____

2 _____

3 _____

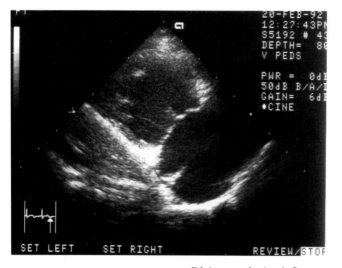
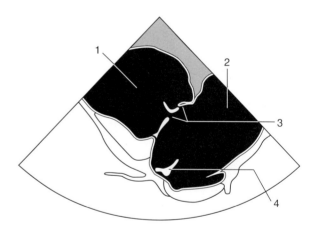

Right ventricular inflow tract, long axis, systolic image.

1 _____   3 _____

2 _____   4 _____

Figure 22-32.

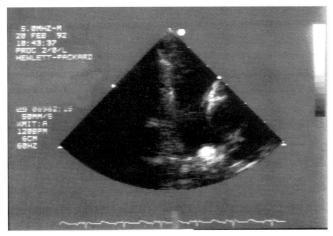 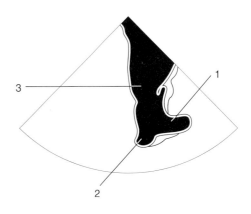

Right ventricular outflow tract, parasternal long axis, systolic image.

1 _____

2 _____

3 _____

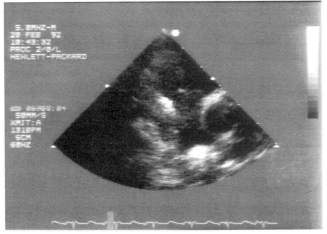 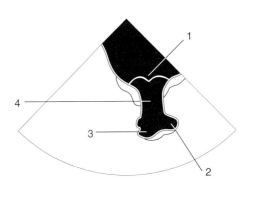

Right ventricular outflow tract, parasternal long axis, diastolic image.

1 _____   3 _____

2 _____   4 _____

Figure 22-33.

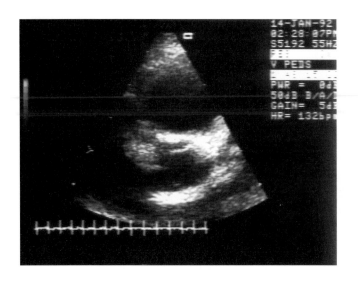
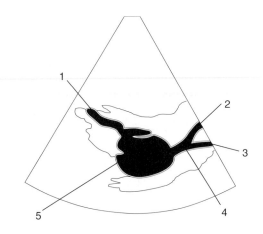

1 _____   4 _____

2 _____   5 _____

3 _____

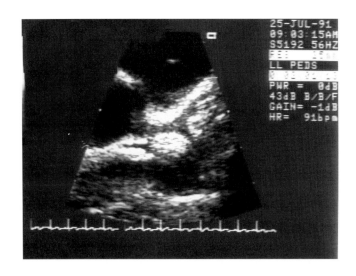
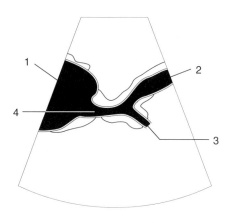

1 _____   3 _____

2 _____   4 _____

Proximal coronary arteries as they exit the aorta.

Figure 22–34.

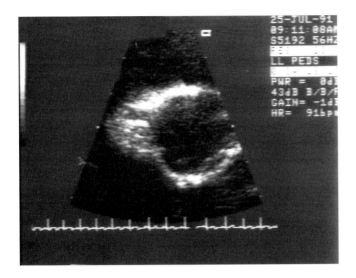
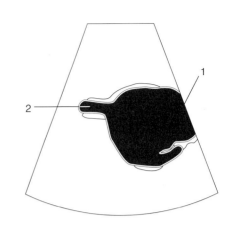

1 _____

2 _____

Proximal coronary artery exiting the aorta.

Figure 22–34. *Continued*

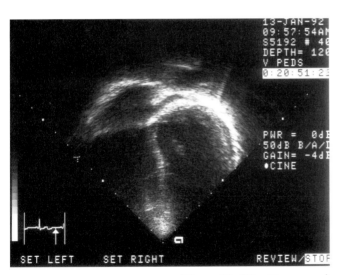
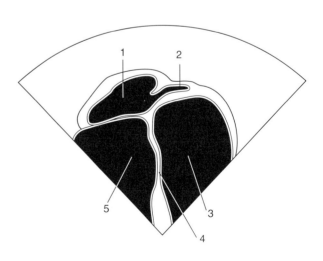

Figure 22–35. Coronary sinus apical four chamber section.

1 _____   4 _____

2 _____   5 _____

3 _____

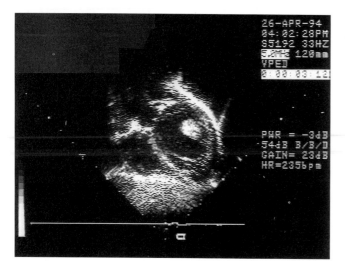
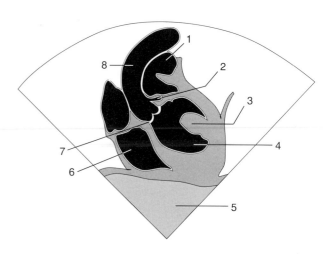

Heart sagittal section.

1 _____   5 _____

2 _____   6 _____

3 _____   7 _____

4 _____   8 _____

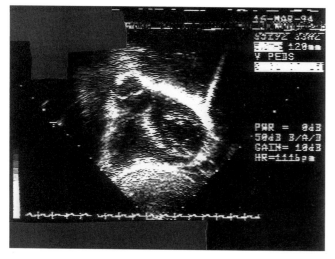
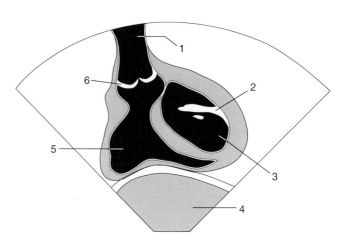

Heart short axis section.

1 _____   4 _____

2 _____   5 _____

3 _____   6 _____

Figure 22-36.

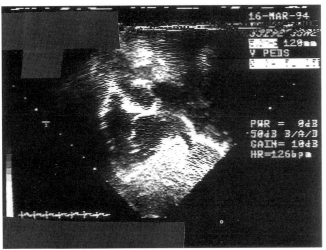
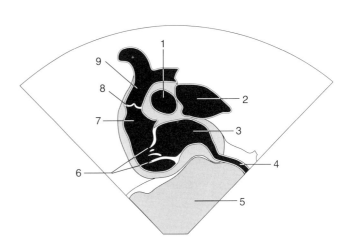

Heart short axis section.

1 _____   6 _____

2 _____   7 _____

3 _____   8 _____

4 _____   9 _____

5 _____

Figure 22–36. *Continued*

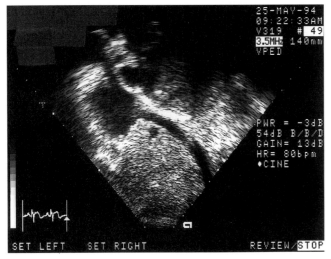 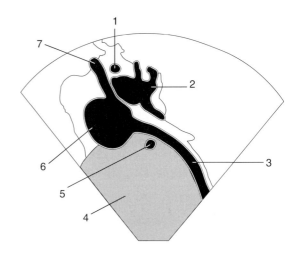

Figure 22–37. Heart subxiphoid section.

1 _____   5 _____

2 _____   6 _____

3 _____   7 _____

4 _____

Chapter 23

ADULT ECHOCARDIOGRAPHY

REVIEW QUESTIONS

1. The anterior surface of the heart is made up almost entirely of the

a. left ventricle

b. right ventricle

c. left atrium

d. right atrium

e. aorta

2. All of the following are found in the right atrium except the

a. Chiari network

b. superior vena cava

c. coronary sinus

d. eustachian valve

e. moderator band

3. The interventricular septum runs continuous with the

a. posterior aortic root

b. anterior aortic root

c. posteromedial papillary muscle

d. posterior mitral valve leaflet

e. anterior mitral valve leaflet

4. All of the following are true about the mitral valve except

a. it is a bicuspid valve

b. the valve is open in diastole and closed in systole

c. the mitral valve helps to control the flow of oxygenated blood in the left heart

d. the mitral valve is a semilunar valve that controls blood flow from the left atrium to the left ventricle

e. the valve leaflets are the anterior and posterior leaflets

5. Normally the dominant pacemaker of the heart is the

a. Purkinje fibers

b. bundle of His

c. AV node

d. SA node

e. electrical impulse

6. Atrial contraction corresponds to which portion of the ECG?

a. P wave

b. Q wave

c. R wave

d. S wave

e. T wave

7. Left heart circulation is as follows

a. pulmonary veins, left atrium, tricuspid valve, left ventricle, aortic valve

b. pulmonary veins, LA, mitral valve, LV, AV

c. pulmonary artery, LA, MV, LV, AV

d. pulmonary artery, LA, TV, LV, AV

e. none of the above

8. The right atrium can be seen in all of the following views except the

a. parasternal long axis

b. parasternal short axis (AV level)

c. apical four chamber

d. subxiphoid four chamber

9. The aortic arch is visualized from which orientation?

a. parasternal

b. apical

c. subxiphoid

d. suprasternal

e. right parasternal

10. Where should the left atrium be measured on the M-model?

a. Q wave

b. midsystole

c. T wave

d. largest dimension

e. QRS complex

11. Normal flow across the aortic valve appears as

a. flow toward the transducer, in the shape of a bullet during systole

b. flow away from the transducer, in the shape of a bullet during systole

c. flow toward the transducer, in the shape of letter "M" during systole

d. flow away from the transducer, in the shape of letter "M" during diastole

e. flow away from the transducer, in the shape of a bullet during diastole

12. Which point on the image shown below corresponds to atrial contraction?

a. D point

b. E point

c. F point

d. A point

e. C point

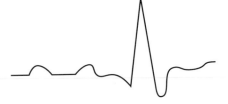
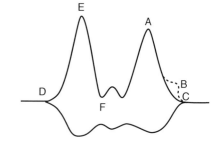

13. Name the view shown below

a. parasternal long axis

b. parasternal short axis (mitral level)

c. right ventricular inflow view

d. apical two chamber

e. apical long axis

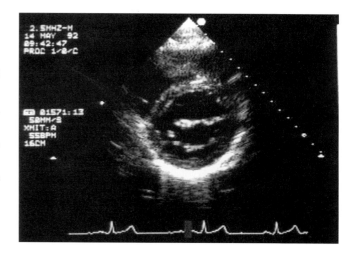

14. Which structure is seen posterior to the aortic root in the image shown below

a. left atrium

b. right atrium

c. left ventricle

d. right ventricle

e. pulmonary artery

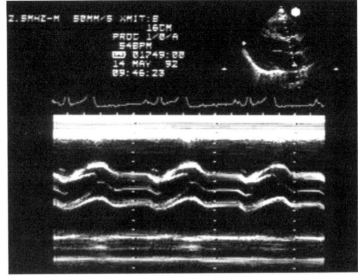

15. Label the structures in the image shown below

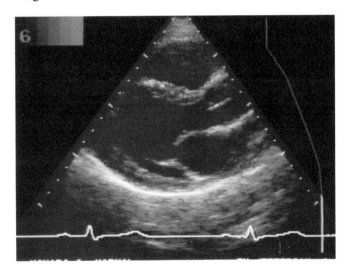

Identify the structures indicated in the following illustrations. These figures duplicate those found in **ULTRASONOGRAPHY: Introduction to Normal Structure and Functional Anatomy**. Refer to the textbook if you need help.

1 _____	13 _____
2 _____	14 _____
3 _____	15 _____
4 _____	16 _____
5 _____	17 _____
6 _____	18 _____
7 _____	19 _____
8 _____	20 _____
9 _____	21 _____
10 _____	22 _____
11 _____	23 _____
12 _____	24 _____

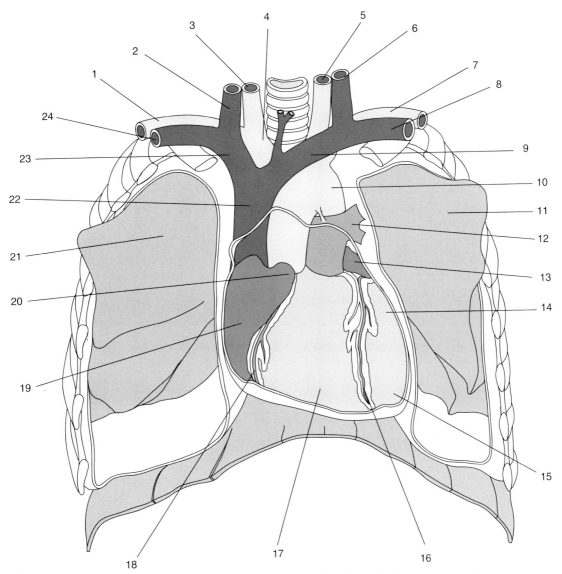

Figure 23–1. External structures and location of the heart in the thoracic cavity.

1 _____   16 _____
2 _____   17 _____
3 _____   18 _____
4 _____   19 _____
5 _____   20 _____
6 _____   21 _____
7 _____   22 _____
8 _____   23 _____
9 _____   24 _____
10 _____   25 _____
11 _____   26 _____
12 _____   27 _____
13 _____   28 _____
14 _____   29 _____
15 _____

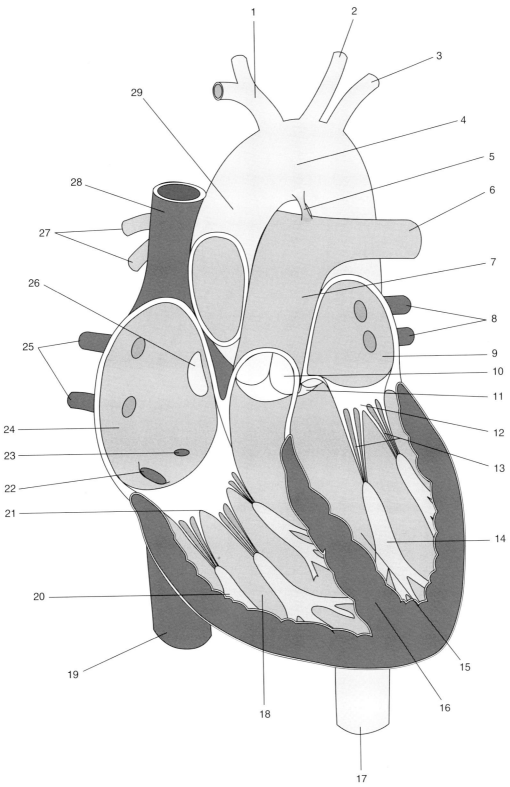

Figure 23-2. Internal structures of the heart.

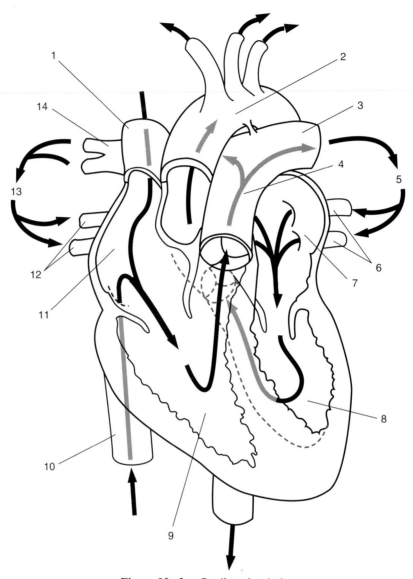

Figure 23–3. Cardiac circulation.

1 _____		8 _____
2 _____		9 _____
3 _____		10 _____
4 _____		11 _____
5 _____		12 _____
6 _____		13 _____
7 _____		14 _____

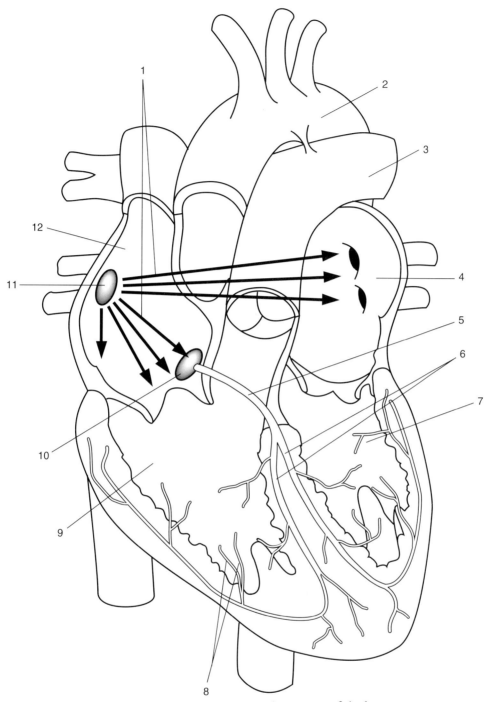

Figure 23-4. Conduction system of the heart.

1 _____   7 _____

2 _____   8 _____

3 _____   9 _____

4 _____   10 _____

5 _____   11 _____

6 _____   12 _____

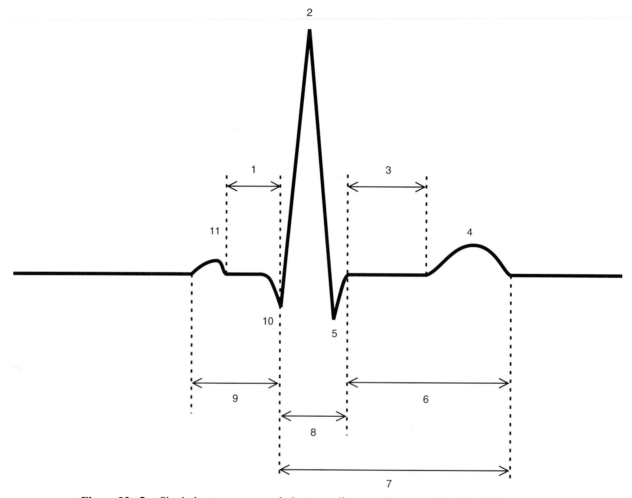

Figure 23–5. Single beat on a normal electrocardiogram demonstrating the QRS complex.

1 _____   7 _____

2 _____   8 _____

3 _____   9 _____

4 _____   10 _____

5 _____   11 _____

6 _____

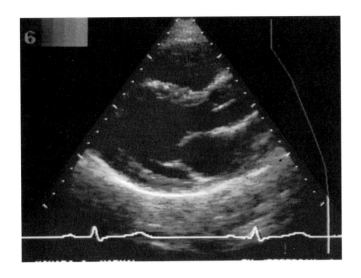
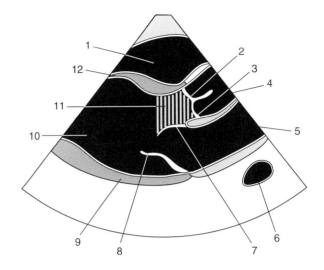

1 _____		7 _____	
2 _____		8 _____	
3 _____		9 _____	
4 _____		10 _____	
5 _____		11 _____	
6 _____		12 _____	

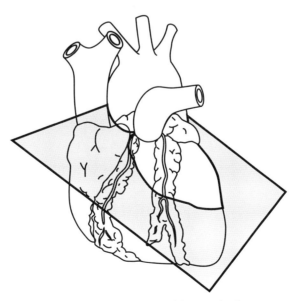

Figure 23–6. Parasternal long axis view.

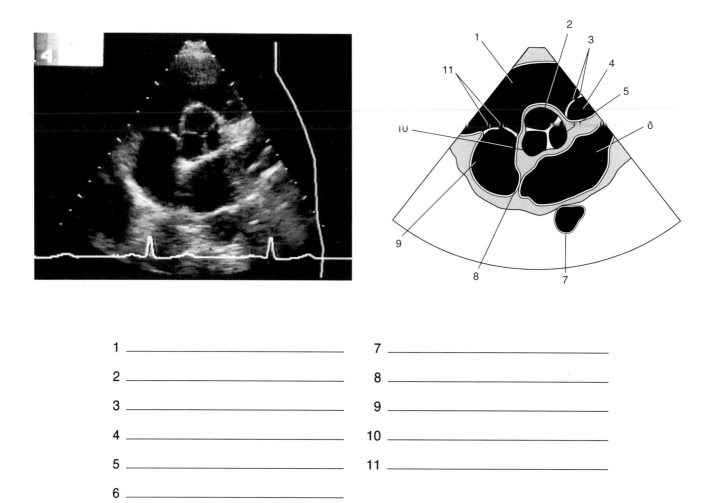

1 _____	7 _____
2 _____	8 _____
3 _____	9 _____
4 _____	10 _____
5 _____	11 _____
6 _____	

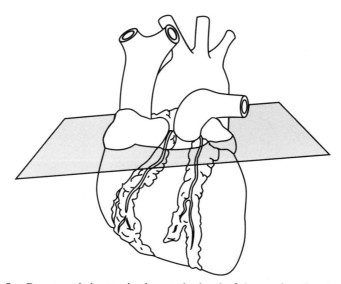

Figure 23–8. Parasternal short axis view at the level of the aortic valve during diastole.

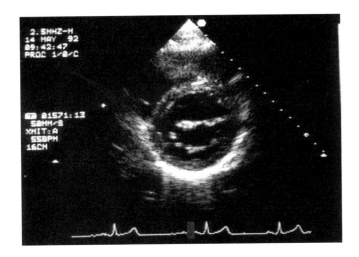
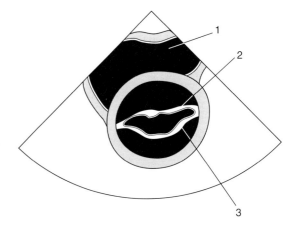

1 _____

2 _____

3 _____

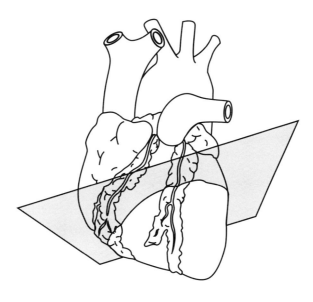

Figure 23–10. Parasternal short axis view at the level of the mitral valve.

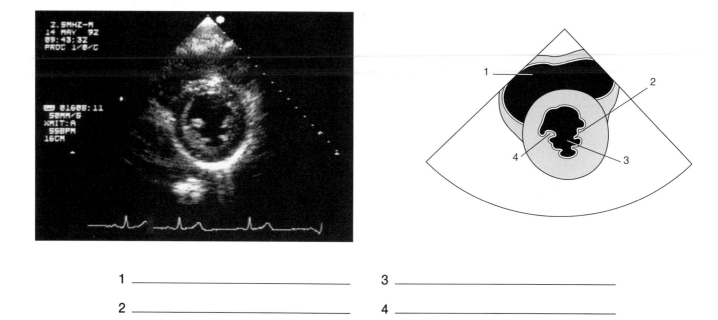

1 _____   3 _____

2 _____   4 _____

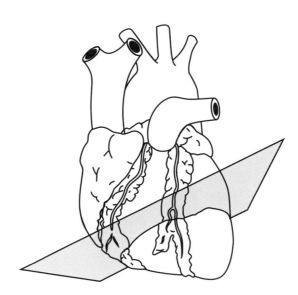

Figure 23-11. Parasternal short axis view at the level of the papillary muscles.

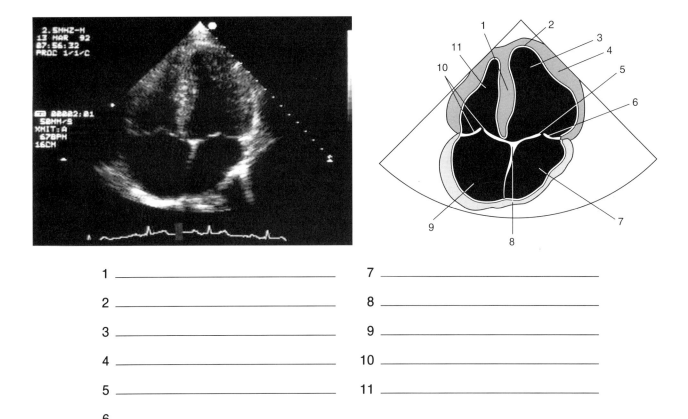

1 _____   7 _____

2 _____   8 _____

3 _____   9 _____

4 _____   10 _____

5 _____   11 _____

6 _____

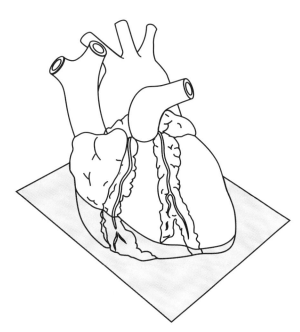

Figure 23–12. Apical four chamber view.

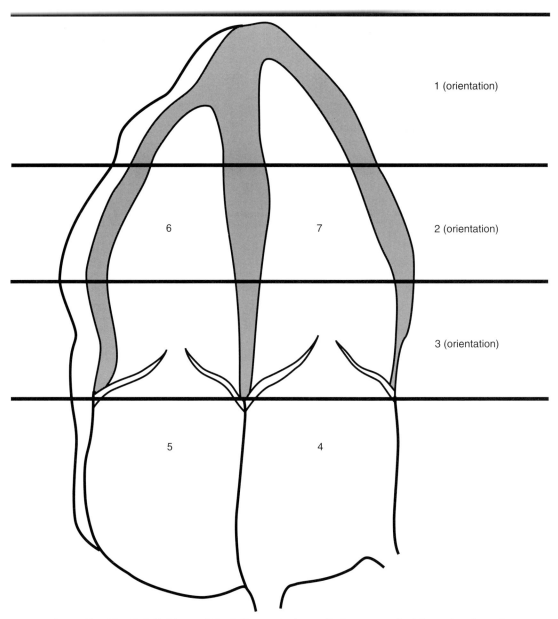

Figure 23–13. Subdivisions of the left ventricular walls from an apical four chamber view.

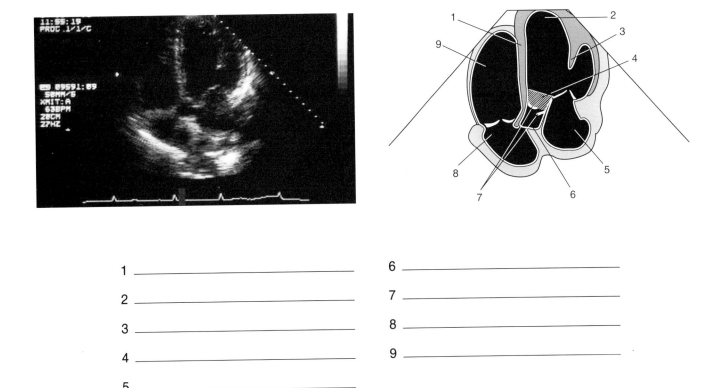

1 _____   6 _____

2 _____   7 _____

3 _____   8 _____

4 _____   9 _____

5 _____

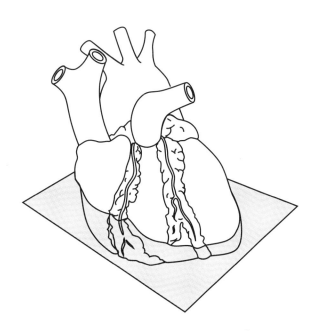

Figure 23-14. Apical five chamber view.

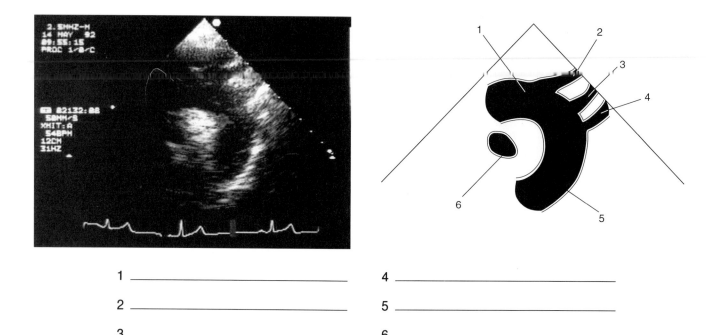

1 _____	4 _____
2 _____	5 _____
3 _____	6 _____

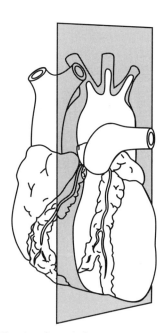

Figure 23-15. Aortic arch from the suprasternal notch.

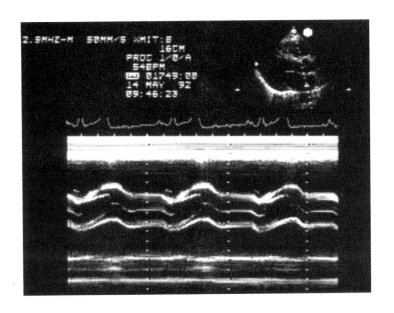

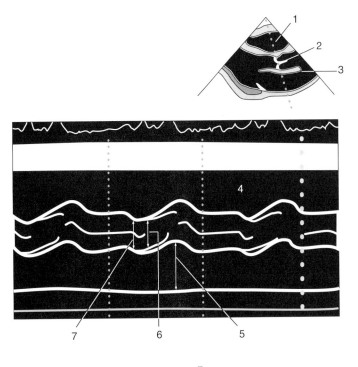

1 _____   5 _____

2 _____   6 _____

3 _____   7 _____

4 _____

Figure 23-17. M-mode at the level of the aortic valve.

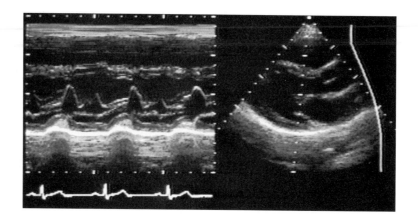

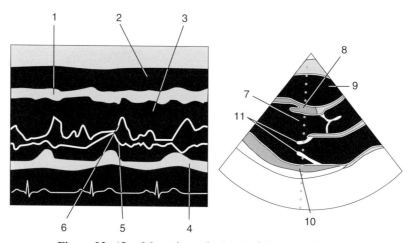

Figure 23-18. M-mode at the level of the mitral valve.

1 _____   7 _____

2 _____   8 _____

3 _____   9 _____

4 _____   10 _____

5 _____   11 _____

6 _____

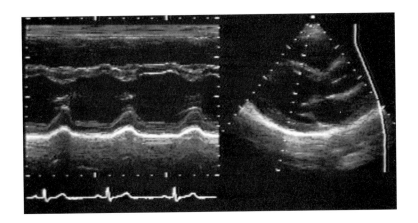

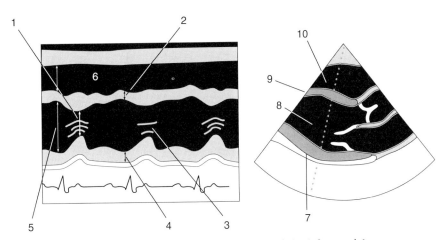

Figure 23-20. M-mode at the level of the left ventricle.

1 _____   6 _____

2 _____   7 _____

3 _____   8 _____

4 _____   9 _____

5 _____   10 _____

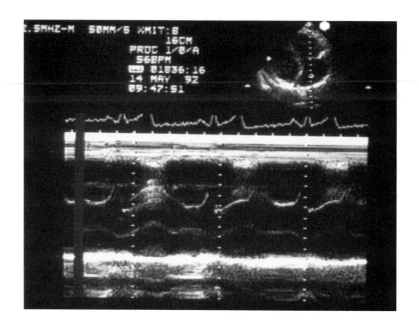

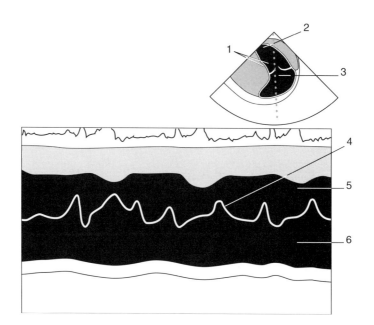

1 _____	4 _____
2 _____	5 _____
3 _____	6 _____

Figure 23–21. M-mode through the tricuspid valve.

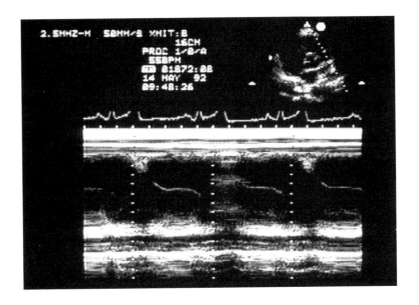

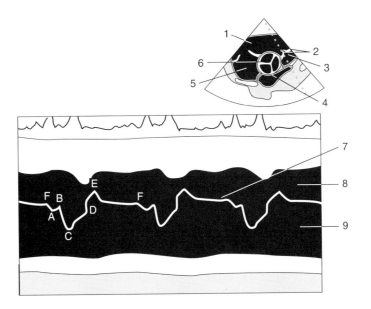

1 _____	6 _____
2 _____	7 _____
3 _____	8 _____
4 _____	9 _____
5 _____	

Figure 23-22. M-mode through the pulmonic valve with its proper alphabetical labels.

Chapter 24

VASCULAR TECHNOLOGY

REVIEW QUESTIONS

1. Indirect vascular laboratory evaluations are best defined as

a. B-mode imaging combined with Doppler velocity spectral analysis

b. tests which examine blood vessels at the site of disease

c. physiologic test procedures which demonstrate pressure and/or volume changes in vessels distal to the location of disease

d. Duplex evaluations which examine the velocity spectral patterns distal to the location of disease

2. Which of the following vessels is not a part of the cerebrovascular system?

a. common carotid artery

b. vertebral artery

c. internal iliac artery

d. internal carotid artery

3. The internal carotid artery supplies the high resistance vascular beds of the brain and eye.

a. true

b. false

4. Which of the following is not a component of the Doppler equation?

a. angle of the Doppler beam with respect to the path of blood flow

b. the speed of sound in soft tissue

c. the Doppler peak diastolic frequency

d. the velocity of blood flow

5. The Doppler time velocity waveform from the normal common carotid artery is characterized by all of the following except

a. rapid systolic deceleration

b. systolic window

c. spectral broadening

d. constant forward diastolic flow

6. Which of the following does not accurately define the left common iliac artery?

a. the vessel lies posterior to the ureter and anterior to the peritoneum

b. the left common iliac vein is posterior to the artery

c. the psoas magnus muscle borders the artery laterally

d. the vessel is the first segment of the peripheral arterial tree distal to the aorta

7. In the absence of peripheral arterial occlusive disease, systolic pressure is greater in the tibial arteries than in the abdominal aorta.

a. true

b. false

8. Which of the following is not a characteristic of a normal peripheral artery?

a. narrow systolic Doppler spectral bandwidth

b. reversed diastolic flow

c. blunted systolic peak

d. systolic window

334

9. Which of the following vessels is not a part of the deep venous system of the lower extremities?

a. profunda femoris vein

b. perforator vein

c. superficial femoral vein

d. anterior tibial vein

10. The gastrocnemius veins are part of the deep venous system and normally empty into the greater saphenous vein of the thigh.

a. true

b. false

11. Which of the following statements is incorrect?

a. venous flow from the legs is under control of the calf muscle pump

b. during exercise, venous pressure at foot level will exceed 40 mm Hg

c. the direction of venous flow is normally from the superficial venous system to the deep venous system

d. veins can withstand tremendous volume change with little change in transmural pressure due to the small amount of elastin found in the venous wall

12. Which of the following statements is incorrect?

a. the inferior mesenteric artery lies anterolateral to the abdominal aorta and enters the pelvis as the superior hemorrhoidal artery

b. the suprarenal abdominal aortic Doppler velocity waveform is triphasic due to the high resistance vascular bed of the fasting superior mesenteric artery

c. the kidneys and liver are high resistance end organs

d. the Doppler time velocity waveform from the postprandial superior mesenteric artery will demonstrate low diastolic flow due to the change in the vascular resistance of the stomach and small intestine that occurs with digestion

13. The Doppler special waveform from the normal renal artery will exhibit constant forward diastolic flow.

a. true

b. false

14. Which of the following is an incorrect statement regarding blood flow to the kidney?

a. the Doppler velocity signal from the interlobar arteries demonstrates significant forward diastolic flow

b. the spectral waveform from the arcuate vessels of the kidney of a patient in chronic renal failure will exhibit decreased diastolic flow

c. due to the high metabolic demands of the kidney, flow is forward during diastole

d. the velocity spectral waveforms from the medulla and cortex of a kidney are normally pulsatile

15. The goal of the vascular diagnostic laboratory is to answer the following questions using an array of indirect and direct noninvasive evaluations: Is vascular disease present? Where is it located? How severe is the disease process? What is the prognosis? Are medical/surgical results being obtained?

a. true

b. false

Identify the structures indicated in the following illustrations. These figures duplicate those found in **ULTRASONOGRAPHY: Introduction to Normal Structure and Functional Anatomy**. Refer to the textbook if you need help.

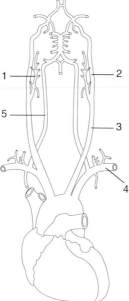

Figure 24-1. The extracranial cerebrovascular system.

1 _____   4 _____

2 _____   5 _____

3 _____

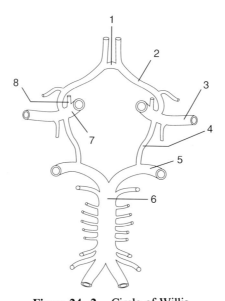

Figure 24-2. Circle of Willis.

1 _____   5 _____

2 _____   6 _____

3 _____   7 _____

4 _____   8 _____

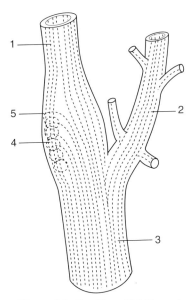

Figure 24–7. Carotid bifurcation.

1 _____

2 _____

3 _____

4 _____

5 _____

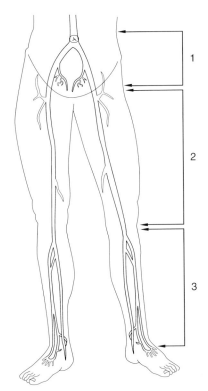

Figure 24–12. Lower extremity peripheral arterial tree.

1 _____

2 _____

3 _____

From Neumyer MM, Thiele BL: The evaluation of lower extremity occlusive disease with Doppler ultrasonography. In Taylor KJW, Burns PN, Wells PNT (eds.): Clinical Applications of Doppler Ultrasound, New York, Raven Press, 1988.

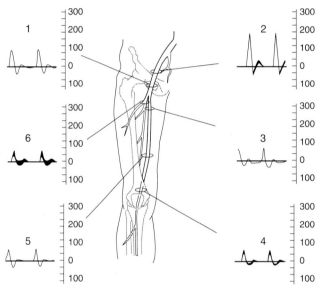

Figure 24-18. Normal velocity spectral waveforms.

1 _____   4 _____

2 _____   5 _____

3 _____   6 _____

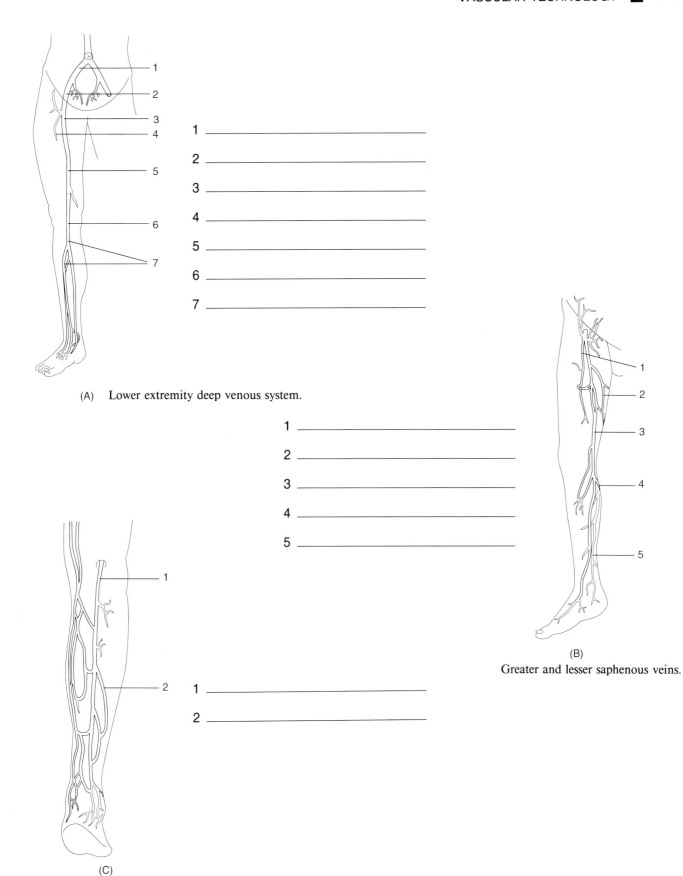

(A)   Lower extremity deep venous system.

1 _____

2 _____

3 _____

4 _____

5 _____

6 _____

7 _____

1 _____

2 _____

3 _____

4 _____

5 _____

(B)
Greater and lesser saphenous veins.

(C)
Greater and lesser saphenous veins.

1 _____

2 _____

Figure 24–19.

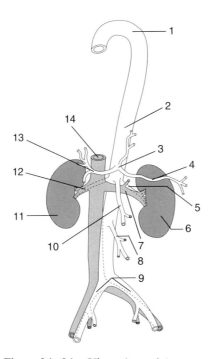

Figure 24–24. Visceral arterial system.

1 _____	8 _____
2 _____	9 _____
3 _____	10 _____
4 _____	11 _____
5 _____	12 _____
6 _____	13 _____
7 _____	14 _____

Chapter 25

INTRODUCTION TO ULTRASOUND OF HUMAN DISEASE

REVIEW QUESTIONS

1. The organ shown below would best be described by which term?

a. cystic

b. homogenous

c. nonhomogenous

d. calcified

2. The image shown below demonstrates which type of pathology?

a. cystic mass

b. solid mass

c. complex mass

d. calcified structure

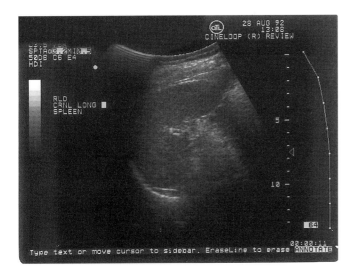

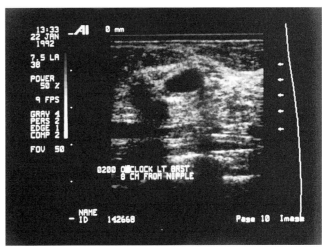

Image courtesy of Acoustic Imaging, Inc., Phoenix, AZ.

3. The image shown below demonstrates which type of pathology?

a. cystic mass

b. solid mass

c. complex mass

d. calcified structure

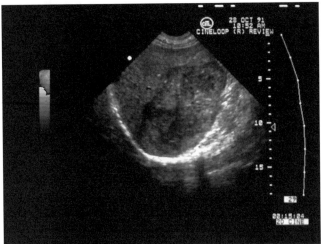

Image courtesy of ATL, Inc., Bothell, WA.

5. The image shown below demonstrates which type of pathological state?

a. cystic mass

b. solid mass

c. complex mass

d. calcified structure

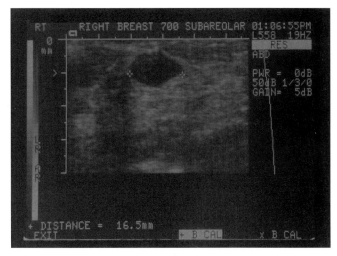

Image courtesy of Acuson Corp., Mountain View, CA.

4. The image shown below demonstrates which type of shadowing?

a. pathological

b. regular

c. refractive

d. none of the above

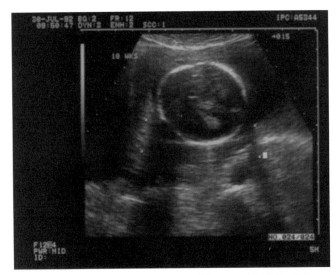

Image courtesy of the Group for Women, Norfolk, VA.

6. Which statement best describes the image shown below?

a. cystic mass with posterior through transmission

b. solid mass with smooth borders

c. mixed echogenically solid mass with irregular borders

d. isoechoic solid mass with irregular borders

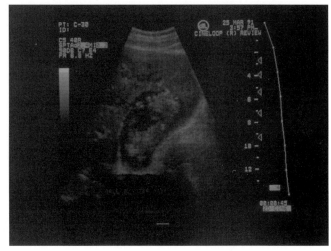

Image courtesy of ATL, Inc., Bothell, WA.

7. Which statement best describes the image shown below?

a. cystic mass with posterior through transmission

b. solid mass with smooth borders

c. primarily solid complex mass

d. isoechoic solid mass with irregular borders

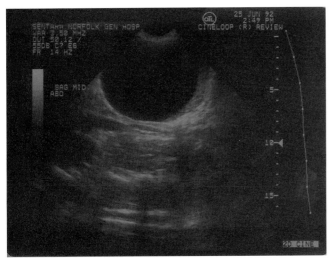

Image courtesy of Sentara Norfolk General, Norfolk, VA.

8. Which statement best describes the image shown below?

a. cystic mass with posterior through transmission

b. solid mass with smooth borders

c. primarily solid complex mass

d. calcific mass with posterior shadowing

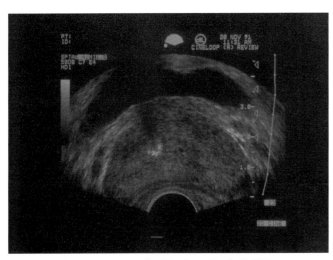

Image courtesy of ATL, Inc., Bothell, WA.

9. Which statement best describes the image shown below?

a. cystic mass with posterior through transmission

b. solid mass with mixed internal echogenicities

c. primarily solid complex mass

d. calcific mass with posterior shadowing

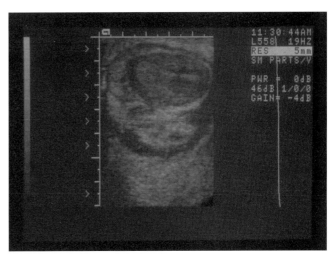

Image courtesy of Acuson Corp., Mountain View, CA.

10. Which of the following statements best describes the typical appearance of a liver containing metastatic tumors?

a. homogeneous texture of medium to high echogenicity

b. homogeneous texture of medium to low echogenicity

c. nonhomogeneous echo texture containing discrete areas of hypoechogenicity

d. multiple masses demonstrating irregular borders and variable echogenicity

e. both c and d may be appropriate

11. A true cyst

a. has smooth walls

b. has no internal echoes

c. may contain anterior echoes

d. has posterior through transmission

e. has all of the above

12. Since it is recommended that sonographers not state a diagnosis when reporting the findings of pathology during an ultrasound examination, it is necessary only for sonographers to be able to recognize textural appearances. It is not important for them to be familiar with the pathological processes associated with the area of interest.

    a. true

    b. false

13. Which of the following statements is correct?

    a. solid masses may have variable echogenicity

    b. all cystic masses have smooth borders

    c. complex masses are never found in conjunction with adjacent vasculature

    d. posterior through transmission occurs because very little sound passes through a mass

14. Ultrasound is able to definitively identify all pathological processes within the abdomen.

    a. true

    b. false

Match the following

15. decreased echogenicity _____

16. posterior through transmission _____

17. posterior shadowing _____

18. mixed echogenicity _____

19. septation _____

    a. complex mass

    b. increased echogenicity posterior to a mass

    c. thin membranous component within a cystic mass

    d. hypoechoic

    e. anechoic area posterior to a calcific mass with clean borders

20. All posterior shadowing arises from pathological conditions.

    a. true

    b. false

Identify the structures indicated in the following illustrations. These figures duplicate those found in **ULTRASONOGRAPHY: Introduction to Normal Structure and Functional Anatomy**. Refer to the textbook if you need help.

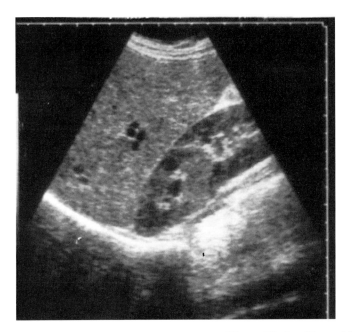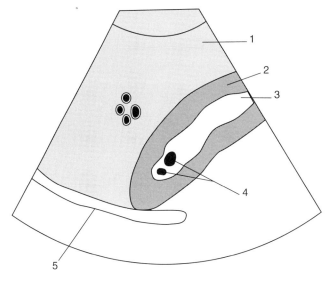

Figure 25-1. Normal liver and right kidney.

1 _____   4 _____

2 _____   5 _____

3 _____

Image courtesy of Acuson Corp., Mountain View, CA.

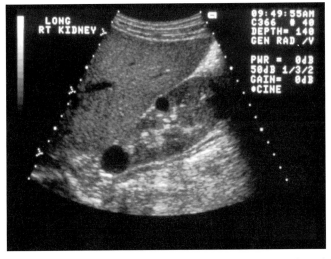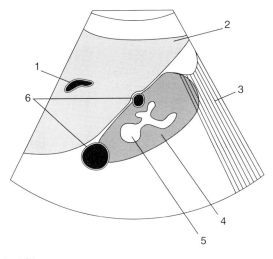

Figure 25-2. Liver and right kidney.

1 _____   4 _____

2 _____   5 _____

3 _____   6 _____

Image courtesy of Sentara Norfolk General Hospital, Norfolk, VA.

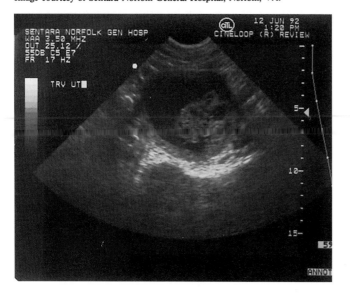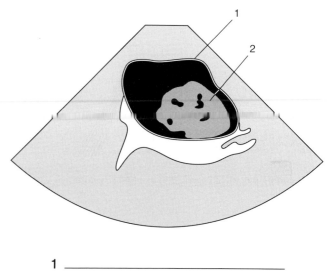

1 _____

2 _____

Image courtesy of Acuson Corp., Mountain View, CA.

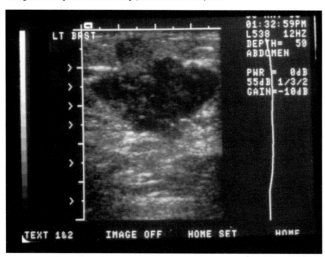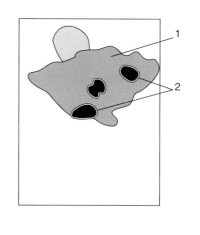

1 _____

2 _____

Figure 25–3. Complex masses.

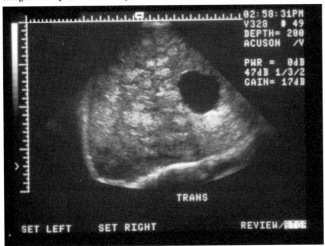

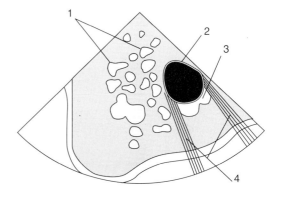

Liver mass.

1 _____

2 _____

3 _____

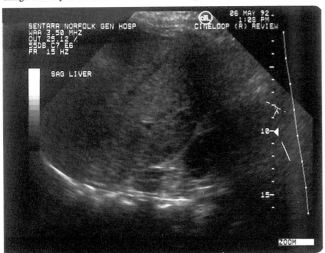

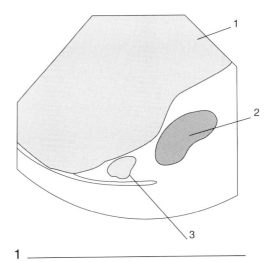

Adrenal gland mass.

1 _____

2 _____

3 _____

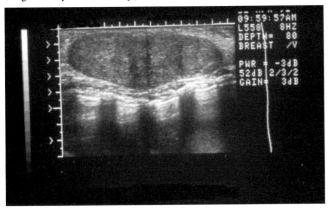

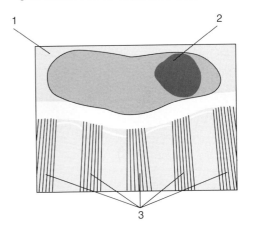

Breast mass.

Figure 25–4.

1 _____

2 _____

3 _____

347

Image courtesy of Acuson Corp., Mountain View, CA.

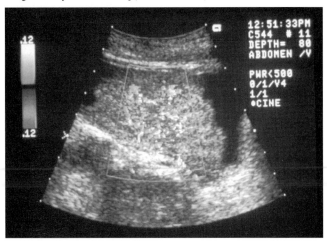
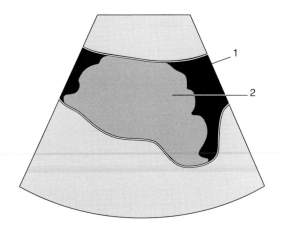

Figure 25-5. Bladder mass.

1 _____

2 _____

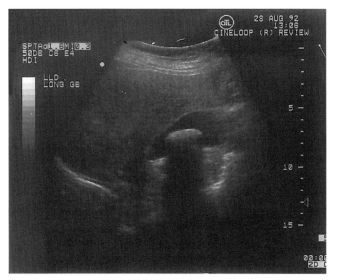
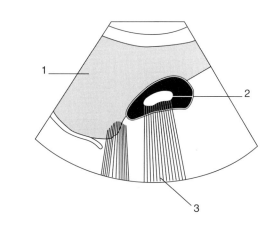

Figure 25-6. Gallstone.

1 _____

2 _____

3 _____

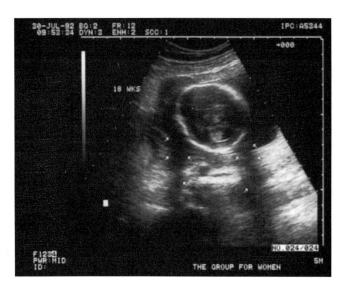
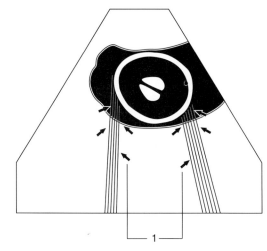

Figure 25-7. Fetal skull.

1 _____

ANSWERS

CHAPTER 1

1.	b	17.	a	33.	d	49.	b
2.	a	18.	a	34.	d	50.	d
3.	a	19.	b	35.	a	51.	a
4.	d	20.	d	36.	b	52.	b
5.	c	21.	a	37.	c	53.	c
6.	b	22.	b	38.	c	54.	c
7.	b	23.	c	39.	b	55.	b
8.	b	24.	c	40.	d	56.	c
9.	c	25.	a	41.	b	57.	b
10.	a	26.	a	42.	c	58.	d
11.	a	27.	b	43.	c	59.	a
12.	d	28.	d	44.	b	60.	d
13.	c	29.	d	45.	c	61.	d
14.	b	30.	c	46.	d	62.	b
15.	c	31.	c	47.	b	63.	d
16.	c	32.	a	48.	c	64.	c
						65.	c

CHAPTER 2

1.	c	5.	c	9.	b	13.	c
2.	c	6.	b	10.	c	14.	d
3.	a	7.	d	11.	b	15.	c
4.	d	8.	a	12.	a		

CHAPTER 3

1.	d	6.	d	11.	a	16.	b
2.	b	7.	d	12.	b	17.	c
3.	d	8.	a	13.	d	18.	c
4.	b	9.	c	14.	c	19.	d
5.	a	10.	b	15.	a	20.	c

CHAPTER 4

1. b. The pancreas is a retroperitoneal organ.

2. a. The gallbladder is an intraperitoneal organ.

3. c. The left renal vein lies transversely as it runs from the kidney to the inferior vena cava.

4. c. The portal vein lies in a transverse oblique position.

5. d. Medial—the anatomic areas appreciated on a sagittal section are anterior, posterior, superior, inferior.

6. c. Anterior—the anatomic areas appreciated on a coronal section are lateral, medial, superior, inferior.

7. a. Superior—the anatomic areas appreciated on a transverse section are anterior, posterior, right lateral, left lateral from either an anterior or posterior approach, or lateral, medial, anterior, posterior from either a right lateral or left lateral approach.

8. d. The location of the transducer and sound wave approach.

9. b. Sonographic appearance—the size, shape, and adjacent relationships of structures is the same on an ultrasound image section and the cadaver section.

10. b. Annular array is a type of ultrasound transducer.

11. a. Inferior (refer to anatomy layering figures).

12. b. Lateral (refer to anatomy layering figures).

13. b. Posterior (refer to anatomy layering figures).

14. c. Right lateral (refer to anatomy layering figures).

15. c. Pancreas neck and the uncinate process (refer to anatomy layering figures).

CHAPTER 5

1. a	9. d	17. a, d	25. d
2. c	10. b	18. c	26. a
3. b	11. d	19. d	27. c
4. c	12. c	20. b	28. b
5. d	13. c	21. c	29. c
6. a	14. a	22. c	30. a
7. c	15. b	23. a	
8. b	16. d	24. b	

CHAPTER 6

1. c. The gallbladder lies in the gallbladder fossa located on the posterior and inferior portion of the right lobe of the liver.

2. b. The porta hepatis is a fissure on the visceral surface of the liver where the portal vein and the hepatic artery enter and the hepatic ducts leave.

3. a. The proximal portion of the biliary duct is the common hepatic duct.

4. d. The right and left hepatic ducts are intrahepatic.

5. a. The distal portion of the biliary duct is the common bile duct.

6. c. The portal triad consists of the portal vein, hepatic artery, and common bile duct.

7. c. Normal biliary duct diameter is 1 mm to 7 mm.

8. b. 3 mm or less is normal for gallbladder wall thickness.

9. d. The fundus of the gallbladder is usually just anterior to the superior pole of the right kidney.

10. b. The sonographic appearance of the bile-filled biliary system is anechoic with echogenic walls.

CHAPTER 7

1. Head (bordered by the inferior vena cava and superior mesenteric vein); Neck (bordered by the superior mesenteric vein); Body (bordered by the superior mesenteric artery and splenic vein; Tail (bordered by the splenic vein).

2. Head (pancreaticoduodenal arteries, pancreatic arcade, gastroduodenal artery); Body and Tail (splenic artery branches, specifically, dorsal pancreatic, pancreatica magna, caudal pancreatic arteries).

3. Trypsin (protein); Amylase (carbohydrates); Lipase (fats).

4. Insulin (changes glucose to glycogen); Glucagon (changes glycogen back to glucose); Somatostatin (inhibits alpha and beta cells).

5. The gastroduodenal artery and common bile duct appear as two small, anechoic areas in the head of the pancreas. The gastroduodenal artery is more anterior than the common bile duct. Both vessels appear circular on transverse images, elongated on sagittal images.

6. The pancreas appears more echodense than the liver, but is less homogeneous.

7. Longitudinal. Transverse images show the long axis of the pancreas.

8. The body of the pancreas.

9. The uncinate process.

10. The common bile duct and duct of Wirsung (main pancreatic duct) usually enter the ampulla of the duodenum together. The accessory duct (duct of Santorini) enters the duodenum approximately 2 cm superior to the main duct and common bile duct.

CHAPTER 8

1. The urinary system maintains the body's chemical equilibrium through the excretion of urine, a waste product. Other functions include detoxifying the blood, regulating blood pressure, and maintaining the proper balance of pH, minerals, iron, and salt levels in the blood.

2. The kidneys are anterior to the diaphragm and the psoas, quadratus lumborum, and transversus muscles.

3. The right kidney is posterior to the right lobe of the liver, right adrenal gland, second part of the duodenum, hepatic flexure of the colon, and the jejunum or ileum of the small intestine.

4. The left kidney is posterior to the tail of the pancreas, the left adrenal gland, the spleen and splenic vein, the jejunum, the stomach, and the splenic flexure of the colon.

5. The ureters are retroperitoneal structures that extend inferiorly along the psoas muscle to the urinary bladder. The duodenum, terminal ileum, and right colic, ileocolic, and gonadal (testicular or ovarian) vessels are anterior to the right ureter. The colon and the left colic and left gonadal vessels are anterior to the left ureter. The abdominal portions of both ureters pass anterior to the psoas muscle and bifurcation of the common iliac arteries. The pelvic portions of the ureters pass posterior to the ductus deferens in the male and uterine artery in the female.

6. The urinary bladder is retroperitoneal and lies posterior to the symphysis pubis. The male urinary bladder is anterior to the seminal vesicles and rectum, and superior to the prostate gland. The female urinary bladder is anterior to the vagina, posterior cul-de-sac, and rectum.

7. Normal sizes of urinary system structures are:
Adult kidney: 9–12 cm in length, 4–6 cm in width, 2.5–4 cm in depth
Ureters: 28–34 cm in length, 6 mm in width
Distended urinary bladder wall: 3–6 mm
Female urethra: 4 cm in length
Male urethra: 20 cm in length

8. The formation of urine begins when blood enters the kidney through the renal artery, which branches into interlobar arteries; these in turn branch into afferent arterioles which carry blood into the glomerulus of the nephron, the functional unit of the kidney. The glomerulus filters the blood. Waste is excreted in the form of urine, and useful substances are reabsorbed into the bloodstream.

9. The parts of the urinary system and their sonographic appearance are as follows:
The **true capsule** acts as a protective covering that surrounds the renal cortex. Its sonographic appearance is echogenic.
The **parenchymal cortex** contains the renal cor-

puscle, and the proximal and distal convoluted tubules of the nephron; thus, filtration occurs in the cortex. Its sonographic appearance is homogeneous with medium to low level echoes that are less than or equal to the echogenicity of the normal liver or spleen. The contour of the normal cortex should appear smooth.

The **parenchymal medulla** contains the loop of Henle of the nephron, thus reabsorption occurs there. The medulla consists of eight to 18 medullary pyramids that appear sonographically as triangular, round, or blunted hypoechoic areas to the more urine-filled anechoic areas.

The **arcuate vessels** may be seen sonographically as echogenic dots at the corticomedullary junction.

The **renal sinus** is the central portion of the kidney that contains the minor and major calyces, renal pelvis, renal artery and vein, fat, nerves, and lymphatics. The overall sonographic appearance of the sinus is echogenic because it is surrounded by fat. The renal pelvis and calyces are not seen if collapsed; otherwise they appear anechoic surrounded by the echogenic fat. The renal artery and vein have echogenic walls and anechoic lumina. Unless enlarged, lymph nodes are not seen. Nerves are not yet appreciated sonographically.

The **ureters** are tubular structures that carry urine from each kidney to the urinary bladder. Normal ureters are not generally seen with sonography. However, "ureteral jets"—the effect of the ureter ejecting urine into the bladder—can be seen during real time examination.

The **urinary bladder** is a temporary storage site for urine until it is excreted from the body through the **urethra**. The bladder lumen is not seen sonographically if collapsed; otherwise it appears anechoic. The distended bladder wall appears as a smooth, thin, echogenic line. The urethra, when seen, appears echogenic.

10. Ultrasound is used to evaluate the urinary system for the following reasons:
    renal size
    detection and composition of renal masses and cysts
    urinary system obstruction
    renal abscess
    renal hematoma
    enlarged ureters
    urinary bladder masses
    Doppler evaluation of renal blood flow abnormalities
    sonography-guided biopsies of renal parenchyma or masses
    sonography-guided fluid aspirations
    renal transplant

11. Urinary system normal variants recognized by ultrasound are:
    dromedary hump: localized bulge(s) on the lateral border of the kidney that has the same sonographic appearance as normal renal cortex.
    hypertrophied column of Bertin: an enlarged portion of renal cortex that varies in size and may indent the renal sinus. It has the same sonographic appearance as normal renal cortex.
    double collecting system: occurs when the renal sinus is divided. Each sinus has a renal pelvis. A bifid (double) ureter may also be present. The sonographic appearance is the same as normal renal cortex and sinus.
    horseshoe kidney: occurs when the kidneys are connected, usually at the lower poles. It has the same sonographic appearance as normal renal cortex.
    renal ectopia: occurs when one or both kidneys are found outside the normal renal fossa. Locations include the lower abdominal and pelvic region. Other ectopic locations (e.g., thoracic) are rare.

12. Physicians associated with the urinary system include **urologists**, who specialize in the surgical diseases of the urinary system in women and genitourinary tract in men. The **nephrologist** specializes in medical diseases of the kidney and the **radiologist** specializes in the diagnostic interpretation of imaging modalities that assess renal disease.

13. Diagnostic tests commonly used to evaluate the urinary system include the radiologic examination **IVP (intravenous pyelogram)**, in which a contrast medium (dye) is injected into a vein and x-ray films are taken at specific time intervals to observe kidney function and urinary system anatomy. This test is performed by a radiologic technologist and a radiologist. The examination is interpreted by the radiologist. **CT or CAT scan (computerized axial tomography)** is a radiologic examination in which cross-sectional x-ray images are obtained of the kidneys and other urinary system structures to assess anatomy. A contrast medium may be administered to differentiate between pathology and normal anatomy. This test is performed by a radiologic technologist and a radiologist. The examination is interpreted by the radiologist.

14. The normal laboratory value for **BUN (blood urea nitrogen)** is 26 mg/dl, which represents normal renal function. The normal value for **Cr (creatinine)** is 1.1 mg/dl, which represents normal renal function. Elevations of these values may indicate renal disease.

15. Hormones that affect the kidneys include **aldosterone**, which increases salt and water reabsorption by the kidneys; **renin**, which helps the kidneys maintain blood pressure; and **antidiuretic hormone (ADH)**, which also increases water reabsorption.

CHAPTER 9

1. d	6. b	11. d	16. d
2. b	7. d	12. b	17. a
3. a	8. b	13. d	18. b
4. b	9. c	14. c	19. d
5. d	10. b	15. a	20. c

CHAPTER 10

1. c	10. c	19. a	28. c
2. f	11. b	20. c	29. a
3. a	12. a	21. b	30. e
4. a	13. d	22. d	31. c
5. b	14. b	23. c	32. b
6. c	15. a	24. a	33. d
7. b	16. c	25. b	34. d
8. d	17. b	26. d	35. b
9. a	18. a	27. d	

CHAPTER 11

1. b	4. d	7. c	9. c
2. d	5. a	8. a	10. b
3. a	6. b		

CHAPTER 12

1. a	4. c	7. a	9. a
2. c	5. b	8. b	10. b
3. a	6. a		

CHAPTER 13

1. d	4. a	7. a	9. b (medial and lateral)
2. b	5. a	8. a	10. a
3. a	6. c		

CHAPTER 14

1. True. 46XY is the normal male karyotype while 46XX indicates a normal female.

2. False. Normal seminal vesicles measure approximately 5 cm in length and *less than* 1 cm in diameter. Seminal vesicles measuring greater than 1 cm in diameter are abnormal and should be further investigated for pathology such as obstruction or tumor invasion.

3. a. The ductus epididymis is located within the scrotum, but is not found within the testis.

4. e. The left testicular vein drains into the left renal vein, while the right testicular vein drains into the inferior vena cava. This is important because in the presence of a left varicocele (dilatation of the scrotal veins) the left kidney should be scanned to rule out an obstruction of the left renal vein.

5. c. The ejaculatory ducts are not located within the spermatic cord. Each spermatic cord contains the ductus deferens, testicular arteries, venous pam-

piniform plexus, lymphatics, autonomic nerves, and fibers from the cremaster muscles.

6. True. The peripheral zone accounts for approximately 70% of the normal prostate gland.

7. False. The penis contains two corpora cavernosa and a single corpus spongiosum.

8. c. The body of the epididymis is not seen in the examination of a normal scrotum. The head of the epididymis is normally visualized, but if the body and tail can be visualized, this usually indicates pathology.

9. False. Normal seminal vesicles appear less echogenic (hypoechoic) than the normal prostate.

10. a. The peripheral zone occupies the posterior and lateral portions of the prostate gland and should have a homogeneous echotexture. The other zones cannot be individually distinguished on transrectal ultrasound.

CHAPTER 15

1. c	5. a	9. b	13. b
2. c	6. d	10. a	14. d
3. a	7. b	11. a	15. d
4. c	8. d	12. b	

CHAPTER 16

1. c	4. b	7. d	9. e
2. a	5. c	8. e	10. c
3. d	6. c		

CHAPTER 17

1. d	3. c	5. e
2. c	4. c	6. b

CHAPTER 18

1. c   3. d   5. e
2. a   4. a

CHAPTER 19

1. b   6. b   11. c   15. c
2. d   7. b   12. d   16. a
3. c   8. b   13. b   17. c
4. c   9. b   14. d   18. b
5. b   10. d

CHAPTER 20

1. c   4. e   7. c   9. d
2. b   5. d   8. b   10. d
3. a   6. d

CHAPTER 21

1. a   3. d   5. b   7. a
2. c   4. c   6. d

CHAPTER 22

1. Generally, the heart provides the driving force that propels blood through the vessels for the distribution of nutrients, gases, minerals, vitamins, hormones, and blood cells to the tissues, and for collection of waste products for excretion.

2. The heart is located in the lower anterior chest posterior to the sternum and anterior to the thoracic vertebrae and esophagus. It rests upon the diaphragm in the middle mediastinum, bounded laterally by the right and left lungs; two thirds of the heart lie to the left of the midsagittal plane and one third lies to the right.

3. Blood enters the right atrium from the superior and inferior venae cavae, passes through the tri-cuspid valve and into the right ventricle. From the right ventricle, blood flows through the pulmonary valve into the main pulmonary artery, and into the right and left pulmonary artery branches to the lungs. Oxygenated blood returning from the lungs enters the left atrium from the four pulmonary veins. From the left atrium, blood flows through the mitral valve, into the left ventricle, and out through the aorta to the head and body.

4. The pulmonary circulation is the flow of blood from the right heart to the lungs for oxygenation.

5. The systemic circulation is the delivery of oxy-

genated blood to the head and body from the left heart.

6. The heart muscle has a soft, homogeneous, even-textured echogenicity. The color appears medium to, in some cases, a dark gray. The valves and chordae appear slightly more echogenic than the medium gray heart muscle. The valves appear as thin, flexible linear structures that are freely mobile. The pericardium is the most echogenic structure, with a smooth, white, linear appearance. The cavities, being filled with blood, are black. The left ventricle is shaped somewhat like a bullet (ellipsoid) and the right ventricle more like a triangle. The right atrium should receive the inferior and superior venae cavae. The left atrium should receive four pulmonary veins.

7. The sinoatrial node (SA node) sets the pace of the heart. When the SA node fires, impulses travel through a pathway called internodal tracts to both atria. They immediately contract. As the impulses travel to the atria, they also travel to the atrioventricular node (A-V node). At this point, there is a short delay in activation and transmission. After this delay, the A-V node fires, sending impulses along the bundle of His. From the bundle, impulses move through the Purkinje fibers into the myocardium. The cardiac conduction system enables the heart to produce a synchronous, coordinated, effective heartbeat.

8. The heart is perfused by the coronary arteries. There are a right coronary artery and a left coronary artery. A major branch of the right coronary artery is the posterior descending coronary artery. The left coronary artery divides almost immediately, upon exiting the aorta, into the left circumflex and the left anterior descending coronary artery.

   The heart is drained by the cardiac veins. Generally, they course with the coronary arteries. Most drain into the coronary sinus and empty into the right atrium. The remainder drain directly into the right atrium.

9. Cardiologist.

10. Chest x-ray studies are performed by a radiologic technologist and interpreted by a radiologist. EKG's or ECG's are performed by a technician and interpreted by a cardiologist.

11. The oxygen content in the right side of the heart is normally lower than in the left side. Pressures on the right side (pulmonary circulation) are lower than those on the left side (systemic circulation).

CHAPTER 23

1.	b	5.	d	9.	d	13.	b
2.	e	6.	a	10.	d	14.	a
3.	b	7.	b	11.	b	15.	
4.	d	8.	a	12.	d		

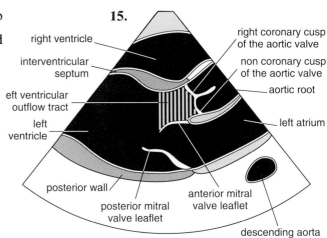

CHAPTER 24

1. b	5. c	9. b	13. a
2. c	6. a	10. b	14. d
3. b	7. a	11. b	15. a
4. c	8. c	12. c	

CHAPTER 25

1. b	6. c	11. e	16. b
2. a	7. a	12. b	17. e
3. b	8. d	13. a	18. a
4. c	9. b	14. b	19. c
5. c	10. e	15. d	20. b

YOUR FIRST SCANNING EXPERIENCE

Betty Bates Tempkin

The primary role of a sonographer is to provide interpretable images for diagnosis by a physician. This goal is totally dependent on the skill of the operator. Becoming an accomplished sonographer happens with practice and the development of good scanning techniques. Starting can be frustrating at times but anything worth doing is not without effort! Informing yourself with established scanning criteria should take the struggle out of scanning while ensuring accuracy, standardization, and quality. To master this skill is to directly contribute to an integral part of patient evaluation.

Before you scan for the first time, review the eight orientation guidelines for learning sectional anatomy in Chapter 4 of the textbook.

Whether you are in a classroom or clinical setting, certain professional and clinical standards should be followed. First, you must be able to properly handle the ultrasound equipment. Practice attaching and detaching transducers from the machine. Be comfortable operating the camera and loading and unloading film cassettes. Experiment with the machine controls to be familiar with their results. (Refer to Chapters 1 and 2 of the text: Physics and Instrumentation, and "Knobology" in the appendix.)

Second, be sure you have the right patient. Check patient identification bracelets and the chart. Introduce yourself and briefly explain the ultrasound examination. Assist the patient in every possible way; always practice safety and be courteous and respectful. Keep conversations professional and never give a patient your opinion of the study or a diagnosis.

Your first scan will be of the abdominal aorta because it is easy to recognize sonographically. It is important at this stage to review the location, gross anatomy, and sonographic appearance of the aorta in Chapter 11 of the text. Also, a valuable exercise is to duplicate with playdough the abdominal layers that include the aorta. Use the layering illustrations from Chapter 4 in the textbook as a guide. Choose one color for arteries, another for veins, and so on. This exercise helps differentiate the intricate relationship of adjacent structures and reinforces the layering concept.

Use a scanning protocol—it ensures that you will be methodical and organized while scanning. Following a scanning protocol is like following a recipe. You take certain steps to achieve a specific goal. The following is a suggested scanning protocol for the abdominal aorta.

A. Patient preparation: the patient should fast for at least 8 hours prior to the examination. This is supposed to reduce the amount of gas in the overlying bowel that can obscure visualization of posterior structures. Even if the patient has recently eaten, you still attempt the examination on the chance that you can evaluate the area of interest.

B. Patient position: the best position is determined by what will produce the optimal view. In this case a supine position is the best approach for evaluating the aorta. Alternatively, the aorta can also be seen from a right or left lateral decubitus, right or left posterior oblique, or with the patient sitting semierect to erect. (See Figure 1–1 for different patient positions.) This should alert you to the fact and advantage that multiple approaches are available for solving imaging needs. Simply put, if it does not work in one position, try another.

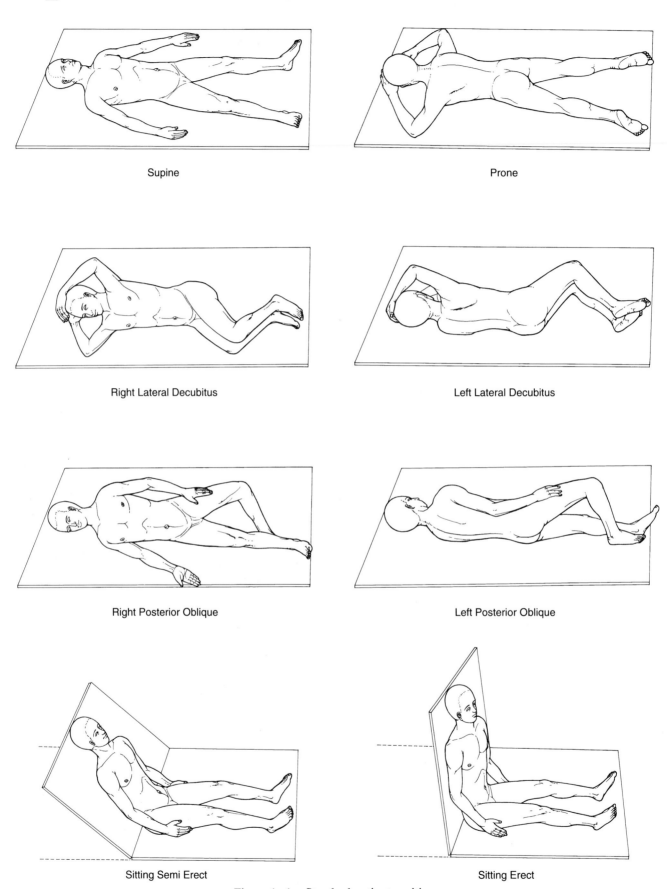

Supine

Prone

Right Lateral Decubitus

Left Lateral Decubitus

Right Posterior Oblique

Left Posterior Oblique

Sitting Semi Erect

Sitting Erect

Figure 1–1. Standard patient positions.

C. Choosing a transducer: you have already learned in Chapter 2 of the text that the higher number megahertz transducers are best for imaging superficial structures and the lower number megahertz transducers are best for evaluating deep structures. Because the aorta is retroperitoneal and one of the deepest structures of the body, the transducer of choice is usually a 3.0 MHz or 3.5 MHz. Try a 5.0 MHz transducer if the patient is very thin. If you are not achieving the desired results with one transducer, switch to another.

D. Breathing technique: respiration causes body structures to move. Deep inspiration forces the diaphragm and everything below it in the abdomen to move down. Deep exhalation causes abdominal structure to move up. You will have to experiment with different breathing techniques to achieve optimal visualization of body structures. The suggested breathing technique for imaging the aorta is normal respiration.

E. The survey: a survey is a detailed comprehensive observation. All ultrasound examinations should begin with a survey of the area of interest and adjacent structures in a least two scanning planes. In the case of abdominal or pelvic structure studies, the entire cavity is evaluated. However, for our purpose of a first scan, we will concentrate only on the aorta. No images are taken during the survey. This is the time to investigate the areas of interest, set technique, and rule out any normal variants or abnormalities.

The longitudinal survey of the abdominal aorta is generally performed first. This is usually from an anterior approach in the sagittal plane. However, the aorta may also be visualized from a left lateral approach in the coronal plane. The steps of the **longitudinal survey** from an anterior approach in the sagittal plane are as follows:

- begin with the transducer perpendicular, at the midline of the body, just inferior to the xiphoid process of the sternum. (See Figure 1–2 for transducer positions and Figure 1–3 for surface landmarks.)

Transducer

Patient's left (LT)

Patient's right (RT)

- slightly move or angle the transducer to the patient's right and identify the distal portion of the inferior vena cava posterior to the liver. You can identify the inferior vena cava by its long, tubular, anechoic appearance and echogenic walls.

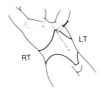

- slightly move or angle the transducer to the patient's left and identify the proximal portion of the aorta posterior to the liver. The aorta can be recognized as a long, tubular, anechoic structure with echogenic walls, differentiated from the inferior vena cava by its anterior branches.

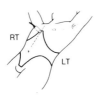

Abbreviation key:
RT (right)
LT (left)
SAG (sagittal)
PROX (proximal)
BIF (bifurcation)
OBL (oblique)
COR (coronal)
TRV (transverse)

Illustrations on this page and to the end of the chapter are taken from Tempkin BB: Ultrasound Scanning: Principles and Protocols. Philadelphia, WB Saunders, 1993.

Perpendicular
The transducer is straight up and down.

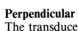

Subcostal
The transducer is angled superiorly just beneath the inferior costal margin.

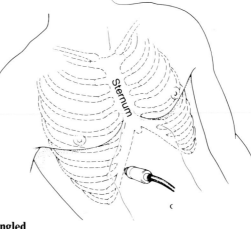

Intercostal
The transducer is between the ribs. It can be perpendicular, subcostal, or angled.

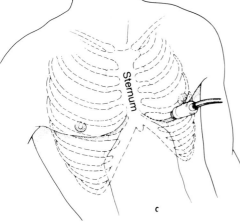

Angled
The transducer is angled superiorly, inferiorly, or right and left laterally at varying degrees.

Figure 1–2. Transducer positions.

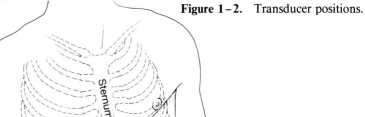

Rotated
The transducer is rotated varying degrees to oblique the scanning plane.

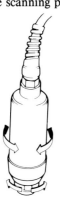

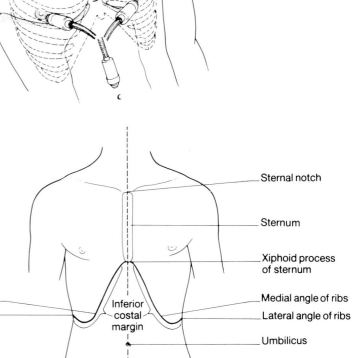

Sternal notch

Sternum

Xiphoid process of sternum

Medial angle of ribs

Lateral angle of ribs

Medial angle of ribs

Lateral angle of ribs

Inferior costal margin

Umbilicus

Symphysis pubis

Figure 1–3. Surface landmarks used as scanning references.

Midline of body (long axis)

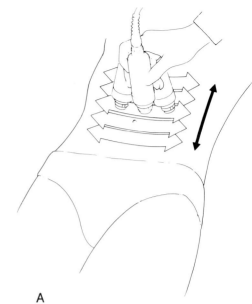

A

Figure 1–4. The rock and slide scanning method. *A*, Rocking side to side while sliding the transducer either superiorly or inferiorly. You can also slide side to side while rocking side to side. *B*, Rocking superiorly and inferiorly while sliding the transducer from side to side. You can also slide superiorly and inferiorly while rocking superior and inferiorly.

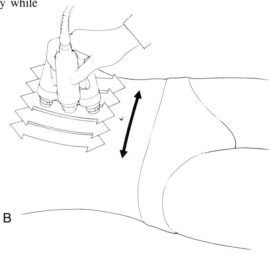

B

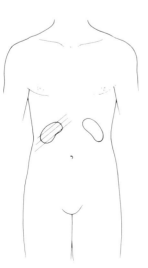

Figure 1–5. Scan according to the lie (or position) of a structure. Rotating the transducer varying degrees obliques the scanning plane to match the position of the structure, giving a more accurate representation.

- while viewing this proximal portion of the aorta, slowly move the transducer inferiorly, using a rock and slide motion. (See Figure 1–4A and B.) Slightly rock the transducer from side to side, scanning through each side of the aorta, while slowly sliding the transducer inferiorly. It may be necessary to rotate the transducer at varying degrees to oblique the scanning plane according to the lie (or position) of the aorta. (See Figure 1–5.) You should be able to see the long axis (full length) of this proximal portion of the aorta and its anterior branches: the celiac axis and superior mesenteric artery.

- continue rocking and sliding the transducer inferiorly through the mid and distal portions of the aorta to the bifurcation (usually at or just beyond the level of the umbilicus).

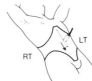

- from the lateral aspects of the most distal portion of the aorta, angle the transducer back toward the aorta and slightly move inferiorly until the bifurcation and common iliac arteries are seen.

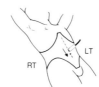

NOTE: alternatively, the bifurcation may be easier to visualize from a left lateral approach in the coronal plane.

- begin with the transducer perpendicular, midcoronal plane, just superior to the iliac crest. Use the inferior pole of the left kidney as a landmark and look for the bifurcation medial, coursing inferiorly. Again, it may be necessary to rotate the transducer varying degrees to visualize the long axis of the bifurcation and the common iliac arteries.

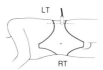

The next step is the **transverse survey** of the aorta. This is usually performed from an anterior approach in the transverse plane. Alternatively, like the longitudinal views of the aorta, the transverse views may also be obtained from a left lateral approach in the transverse plane. The steps of the **transverse survey** from an anterior approach in the transverse plane are as follows:

- begin with the transducer perpendicular, at the midline of the body, just inferior to the xiphoid process of the sternum. (Refer to Figures 1–2 and 1–3.)

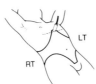

- angle the transducer superiorly until the heart is seen. Slowly, straightening the transducer back to a perpendicular position, look for the aorta just to the left of midline. The aorta will appear round or oval and anechoic with echogenic walls.

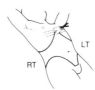

NOTE: alternatively, locating the transverse section of the proximal aorta may be easier by starting from the visualization of the longitudinal portion of the proximal aorta in the sagittal plane. Simply rotate the transducer 90 degrees into the transverse plane visualizing the aorta the entire time.

- while viewing the proximal aorta, slightly rock the transducer superiorly to inferiorly while sliding inferiorly—this way you should never lose sight of the aorta. As you move inferiorly, note and evaluate the aorta's anterior branches: the celiac axis and superior mesenteric artery.

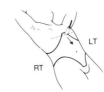

- continue rocking and sliding the transducer inferiorly through the mid and distal portions of the aorta to the bifurcation. As you move inferiorly through the mid portion of the aorta, note and evaluate the lateral branches: the renal arteries.

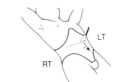

- at the level of the bifurcation, evaluate the proximal portion of the common iliac arteries by scanning through them inferiorly until you lose sight of them. The sonographic appearance of the distal aorta to the common iliac arteries is from a single large round anechoic vessel to two small round anechoic vessels.

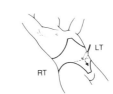

F. Required pictures: ultrasound images reflect isolated sections of structures or samples of the whole. These image sections must clearly represent examples of what was determined during the survey. Like the survey, images have to be documented in two scanning planes. This gives a more dimensional and therefore accurate representation. Furthermore, for legal and clinical standardization the images are labeled to include the patient's name, any identification number, the date, the scanning site, and the initials of the sonographer scanning. Also, the area of interest, the scanning plane, and the transducer megahertz must be part of the film labeling. When endocavital studies are performed, another health professional should witness the procedure and his or her initials should also go on the film.

Remember that the the images you take for the physician should be the best representation for interpretation. It is standard practice to take certain views that give the physician the most information. For example, you survey the entire abdominal aorta from its proximal portion to its bifurcation, but you take only one representative longitudinal and transverse image of each major section. Additionally, for instance, in some institutions the longitudinal image of the proximal aorta must include the celiac and superior mesenteric branches, and the transverse image of the mid aorta must include the renal arteries. While there may be slight variations in protocol according to the interpreting physician, the basic comprehensive images (including those with measurements) should always be the same.

It is also important to note that whenever an image is taken with measurement calipers or any type of labeling directly on the image, that very same image must be taken again without the calipers or labels. This is done for the interpreting physician in case these additions happen to cover some area of interest.

Since the survey of the aorta was done in the sagittal and transverse planes from an anterior approach, the required pictures should be taken in the same manner. The following are the required longitudinal and transverse images of the abdominal aorta and how they should be labeled:

Longitudinal Images/Sagittal Plane/Anterior Approach

1. Longitudinal image of the proximal aorta:

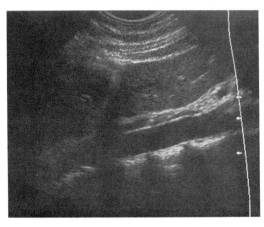 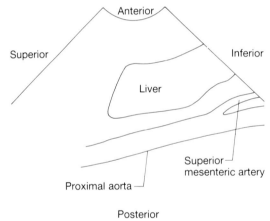

Labeled: AORTA SAG PROX

2. Longitudinal image of the mid aorta:

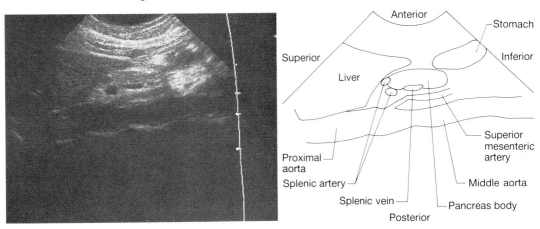

Labeled: AORTA SAG MID

3. Longitudinal image of the distal aorta:

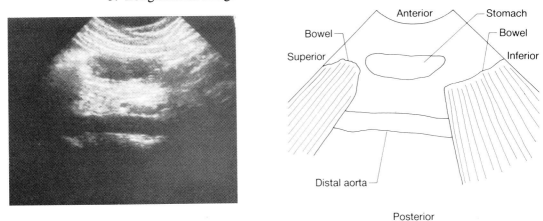

Labeled: AORTA SAG DISTAL

4. Longitudinal image of the aorta bifurcation (common iliac arteries):

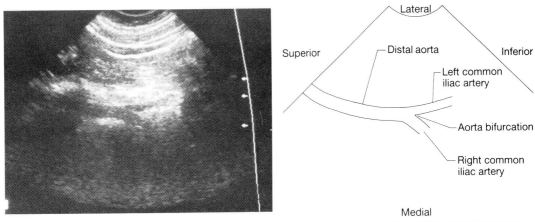

Labeled: AORTA SAG BIF RT OR LT (depending on lateral position of transducer) OR AORTA LT OR RT COR BIF

Transverse Images/Transverse Plane/Anterior Approach

5. Transverse image of the proximal aorta with anterior to posterior measurement (calipers placed on outside wall to outside wall):

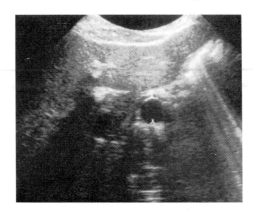

Labeled: AORTA TRV PROX

6. The same image as No. 5 without the measurement calipers:

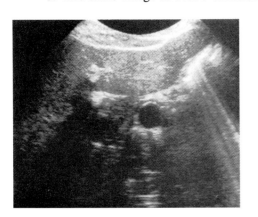
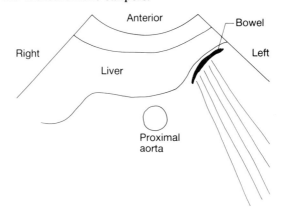

Labeled: AORTA TRV PROX

7. Transverse image of the mid aorta with anterior to posterior measurement (calipers placed on outside wall to outside wall):

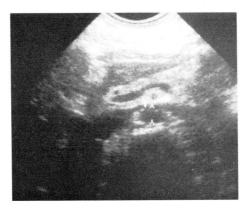

Labeled: AORTA TRV MID

8. The same image as No. 7 without the measurement calipers:

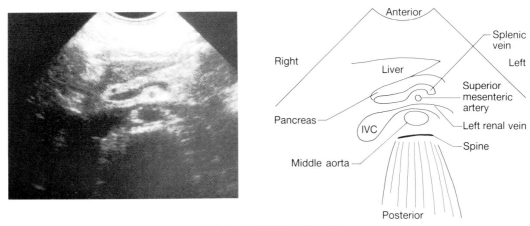

Labeled: AORTA TRV MID

9. Transverse image of the distal aorta with anterior to posterior measurement (calipers placed on outside wall to outside wall):

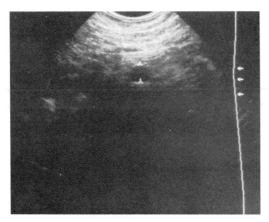

Labeled: AORTA TRV DISTAL

10. The same image as No. 9 without the measurement calipers:

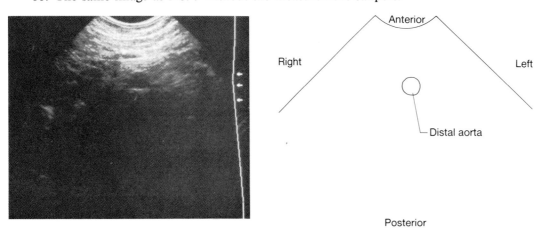

Labeled: AORTA TRV DISTAL

11. Transverse image of the aorta bifurcation (common iliac arteries):

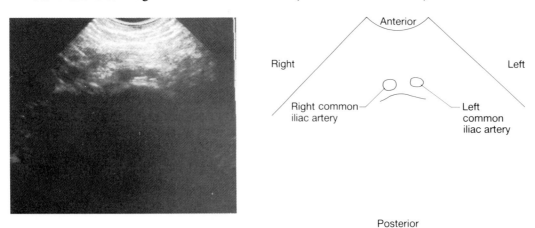

Labeled: AORTA TRV BIF

This sample protocol addresses the basic comprehensive images that should be taken when the abdominal aorta is the area of interest or examination ordered.

Assuming that you have completed Chapter 11 in the text on the abdominal aorta and have a thorough and comfortable understanding of the normal aspects and sonographic appearance of it, keep in mind that if you see something abnormal about the aorta during the survey you must be prepared to evaluate the abnormality and document it. Basically, all abnormalities or pathologies can be evaluated and documented the same way. First, during the survey determine which organ(s) or structure(s) are primarily involved, which if any of adjacent structures are involved, and the composition of the abnormality (solid, cystic, complex, septated, dissected; review Chapter 25, Introduction to Ultrasound of Human Disease, in the text.) The pathology images should follow the standard protocol images and document the clearest representation of the aforementioned, including measurement images in two scanning planes at the greatest dimensions (excluding gallstones, renal stones, hydronephrosis, thrombosis, pleural effusion, or ascites).

The clinical portion of a sonographer's expertise is the most direct and important contribution that a sonographer makes to a patient's ultrasound evaluation. Since this clinical competence is not directly evaluated by registry or licensing, it takes personal initiative and discipline to master these scanning skills. Match the quality of your images with other established protocol images and use feedback from your instructors and/or physicians to monitor your personal progress.

References

1. Tempkin BB: Ultrasound Scanning: Principles and Protocols. Philadelphia, WB Saunders, 1993.